A Collection of My Thoughts (Living with Depression)

Anna Ballard (PhD)

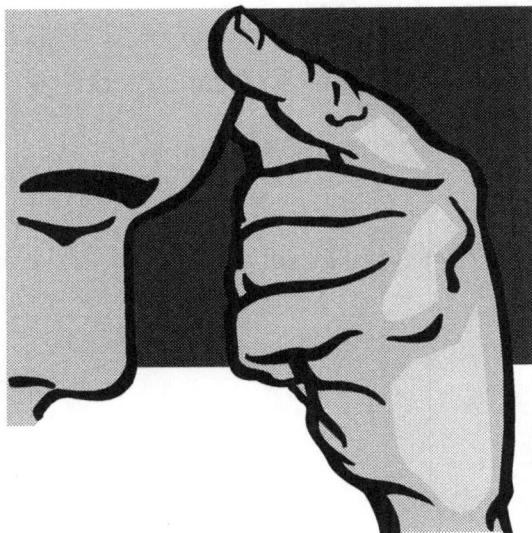

Published by:
Chipmukapublishing
PO Box 6872
Brentwood
Essex
CM13 1ZT
United Kingdom

http://www.chipmunkapublishing.com

Copyright © 2006 Anna Ballard

ISBN 978 1 84747 008 9

ABOUT THE AUTHOR

I was born and brought up in the Vale of Evesham, in the heart of England. As the youngest of four children (I have three older brothers) I was some what spoiled particularly by my father. However, as the youngest I spent my childhood striving to keep up with my siblings and this nurtured a very competitive spirit within me.

In consequence at school this spirit drove me forward and I became a high achiever gaining straight A grades at both O and A level. I was also very fortunate in that I was athletic. To begin with I was a fine swimmer and tennis player reaching county standard in both but when the swimming started to wane I transferred my efforts into canoeing. The village in which I lived had its own canoe club and the opportunities were there for the taking. My canoeing career spanned almost 20 years and I represented my country at four World Championships with my best result being 12th place. Sadly I don't canoe anymore, except recreationally, but in order to satisfy my competitiveness I still play tennis two or three times a week.

During all these years in competitive sport I continued with my academic studies. I attended the University of Birmingham reading Biochemistry and was awarded a 1st Class honours degree followed by my PhD. I also gained two scholarships and received the RT Jones Prize which is awarded to a first year undergraduate who is outstanding in scholarship, personality and contribution to the life of the University as a whole. After University I spent the next 12 years doing medical research mainly looking at mutant strains of Hepatitis B. Again I was very successful as demonstrated by the 15 papers published during that time.

Since 1980 I have been supported by my husband who is himself a canoeing Olympian and who now joins me on the tennis courts. We have two children aged 14 and 11 and we live in a rural area just outside Lichfield to the north of Birmingham.

It was after the birth of my second child that I started to have mental health problems. Firstly I was diagnosed with post natal depression but this soon turned into clinical depression and in 2000 I suffered what you would call a "nervous breakdown". At the time the children were young and demanding plus I was commuting everyday to Nottingham to carry out my research. Eventually something had to give and it was me. I was "sectioned" under the Mental Health Act and detained in hospital for many weeks.

The road to recovery has been a bumpy one but my illness is now well managed with drugs and psychological backup. My research work has been curtailed but I am still employed in a hospital environment and I get a lot of job satisfaction from helping others. Recently I have started to give back to the system from which I have taken so much by sharing the poetry in this book with other people, particularly with those whose lives are touched by mental illness. I hope that what I have done will enlighten and inspire you the reader in the future.

The take home message is one of hope in that for all sufferers of mental illness there is always the possibility of recovery. Of course this may involve taking medication and altering one's perspective of life but eventually a way forward will be found. The poems I have written illustrate how recovery has happened for me and I would like to think that by writing down my experiences I may help others overcome their problems too.

A COLLECTION OF MY THOUGHTS
(LIVING WITH DEPRESSION)

I have composed the book of poetry that follows over the last year (September 2004 to September 2005). In the most part it is a record of the thoughts I have had about life with a particular emphasis on the last 10 years during which time I have suffered with a psychotic depressive disorder. What prompted me to write it was a change in antidepressant (to Venlafaxine) which I believe stimulated the creative part of my brain (the right hemisphere) that wasn't being used before. The effect was quite dramatic and within a week of starting on the new drug I began to churn out my thoughts as poetry. I had never written anything before but what initially started out as a whim rapidly turned into something more substantial. At my peak I was composing one or two poems a day but this has now moderated and I only write when something new happens in my life that I want to document.

Not surprisingly many of the poems centre on mental illness and related subjects. The idea is to lead you on a journey from the depths of despair, through mental illness itself, to help, recovery and rebuilding your life, followed by love and finally general life observations. As a result the poems at the beginning are rather disturbing since they deal with the dark side of mental illness, but don't be put off it is not all doom and gloom. In fact I hope that I have set things down in a way that is both enlightening and maybe even inspiring.

If you want to give me feedback I can be contacted as follows

Write to me care of Chipmunkapublishing ltd

This book is dedicated to my husband and my children

Contents

Preface

If I were to write my life story
Some of it would be rather gory
For though I have achieved great things
Part of it has been depression tinged
I had a wonderful carefree childhood
With loving parents who were kind and good
I did really well at school
Where I gained qualifications of the highest level
Next I tackled University
Reaching even greater heights with a PhD
Medical research then beckoned
And I was able to answer many difficult questions
While doing all this I also excelled in sport
I represented my country and enjoyed the glory that it
brought
I soon became married and had a baby
And later added a second to complete my family
It was at this time that things began to fall apart
I suffered from post natal depression at the start
That then recurred as clinical depression
And ultimately lead me to hospitalisation
At that time I thought it would be better
For me to leave this world altogether
Thankfully I never managed to commit suicide
Because I wouldn't be here with you otherwise
It has taken a long time for me to recover
By taking medication and talking to others
My illness has eventually come under control
And for this small mercy I am thankful
I still have my ups and downs
But I no longer feel the need to frown
My family and friends give me continuous support
They stop me from becoming overwrought
I can now see so many good things that I can do
I am glad to be alive and I hope you feel the same way
too

INTRODUCTION

Just a short message
Before you start to read
The poems at the beginning
Are very disturbing indeed
They are about mental illness
Of which I have first hand experience
Some require a strong stomach
And may touch your conscience
But the rest are purely for entertainment
I hope they make you smile
They are mostly true to my life
So dwell on them a while
It may therefore be better
To start reading from the back
I trust you will digest my scribbling
And give me any feedback
Let me give you a single thought
If I were to have my time again
Even with my ups and downs
I would live it just the same

Mental Illness

If you break your arm
Or you are in a diseased state
Then other people rally round
Because they are able to associate
But if you have a mental illness
This is more difficult to explain
People don't understand
And they can't comprehend your pain
There is nothing to be seen
The problem is locked up in your head
And others shy away
Or just ignore you instead
We need to break down these barriers
And address this subject that's taboo
Because mental illness
Could one day even strike you

Leveller

Mental illness is a great leveller
It hits the rich and the poor alike
You can't predict who will be next
It is indiscriminate about who it strikes
The tramp sitting in the doorway
Or the millionaire in his mansion high
They both could be victims
And you may question why?
It is because anyone can have a faulty brain
Where the right signals aren't getting through
And nobody is to blame
There is nothing you can do
I pray that you never become mentally ill yourself
But if you should then I can tell where to find
The help and support of other sufferers
Who are now further down the line

A Statement

I want to write something profound
A statement that will lift you off the ground
I will say it all in verse
From a point where you can observe
"Having mental health problems
Doesn't mean you are condemned
Just as with any other illness
People do recover, they do get through this
If you suffer or are the one who cares
Then you should be made aware
That the path to normality may be long
But in the end you come out strong
All the introspection that is involved
For the problem to be resolved
Requires you to dig in deep
And find the energy to make recovery complete
Exactly how to do this is difficult to explain
But please remember YOU come back the same

Thoughts

I like to sit and think
Take time to contemplate
Let my thoughts develop
And make my brain pulsate
I can think of abstract things
Or focus on reality
Sometimes my ideas are crazy
But they have meaning to me
Just how do the chemicals in our head
Affect the thought process?
It is a complicated business
Which we do with great success

My message to you

I want to do something special
That will make you really proud
It may be quite outrageous
And make me stand out from the crowd
I want to impart my knowledge
And let others know my thoughts
Maybe I can show them
If they are ready to be taught
'Life is very precious
We should enjoy every minute
We should push back all the barriers
And live it to the limit'
This is the underlying message
That I want to give to you
And you can pass it on to others
So they can share it too

How did I become Depressed?

I didn't just wake up one morning
To find I was depressed
It just crept up on me slowly
In a way I couldn't detect
To begin with it was the little things
That started to go wrong
Although I tried desperately
There was no way of hanging on
I became very irritable
And bad tempered with everyone
But I didn't recognise this
As a prelude to what was to come
I found myself on tenterhooks
All of the time
Waiting for the next disaster

To rock this world of mine
There was also the problem
Of not being able to sleep
This would upset me
And ultimately make me weep
My appetite was affected
I started to pile on the pounds
I was comfort eating
When no one else was around
It was only when I added
All these things together
That it became clear
That life had lost its pleasure
Then I had to illicit
The help of my GP
And I was quickly referred
To the doctor of psychiatry
Now I have professional support
And the proper pills
My problems have been overcome
There has been a cure for my ills

I am about to write some poems
That will lift you up and get you going
But first I must get out of my chair
I must stand up if I am to go anywhere
I will straighten my clothes which are rather staid
And together we will go on an escapade
Through my troubled and murky past
Hopefully to get to the bottom of things at last
Together we will iron out the creases
That have arisen because of my mental illness
We can set the wheels in motion
We don't need a magic potion
And I promise you your view of life will turn
All you have to do is read and learn

CRIES FOR HELP

A Cry for Help

I am ill again
I can see the warning signs
This cancerous depression
Is no more benign
I don't know why it's back
And has raised its ugly head
But I don't want to be here
I would rather be dead
I am in the depths of despair
Feeling sorry for myself
And I am reaching out to you
This is my cry for help

Help Me

Help me because I am dying
I have soldiered on but have now stopped trying
My valiant efforts have been in vain
I haven't managed to rid myself of this infernal pain
My mind gives me such negative vibes
And my life has turned into a rollercoaster ride
I want to jump off and abandon ship
But I am too frightened to actually do it
How can I tell you that all hope is gone?
When you say to me I must carry on
All I want to do is curl up tight in a ball
And pray that you will put an end to it all
Don't leave me here washed up on the shore
Save me from myself before I am no more

Crying

I hang my head down low
I bring my hands up to my face
I can no longer hide my feelings
And the tracks of my tears are easy to trace
But why are you crying?
I hear you exclaim
It is because I am dying inside
And I cannot bear the pain
My soul is disintegrating
And my world is falling apart
There is nothing you can do
I have a broken heart
I am so depressed
All I can do is sit and mope
I have completely given up
I am unable to cope
Here I am in the depths of despair
And I don't think I can carry on
I am looking for a glimmer of light
And some way of hanging on
I turn towards you
As my closest friend
Please help me to move forward
Please make this sorrow end
For now I will stop crying
My energy is all spent
And hope that you are listening
To my strained lament

I Need You

I need you to give me a great big cuddle
Because my life is an uphill struggle
I want your arms to wrap right round
And pull me up from where I was found
I need to feel your warmth beside me
And hope that you are able to guide me
Back to where I should be
Back with the rest of humanity
I have sunk so low into this bottomless pit
That on my own I can't escape from it
I am begging you to rescue me
So that I am not damned for all eternity

The Better of Me

My emotions have got
The better of me
Tears are welling up in my eyes
Can't you see?
For so long I have been
Holding everything back
Trying to conceal my weakness
And pretend I'm immune to attack
Well now I find
I can't cope anymore
I am frightened of the future
And what lies in store
I can no longer hide
Behind my steely façade
I can't keep up this front
In life's game of charades
You believe I am strong
And that I am always composed

But in fact my spirit is broken
My frailty is exposed
Are you my friend
Someone I can rely on?
I trust the answer is 'yes'
Because I need a shoulder to cry on
I am at the end of my tether
I am starting to choke
Please take me in your arms
Before I lose all hope

Prayer

Sometimes I have to say a prayer
In the hope that there is someone there
Who will hear my plight
Even though I know the odds are only slight
I am searching for someone to listen
And who can impart to me their wisdom
For I don't understand
How to take control and be in command
Of my life with all its stress
I need help, I must confess
I look to the Almighty one because
I am completely at a loss
No mortal being can give me the answer
I am looking for some sort of energy transfer
That comes from up on high
And will mend my crumpled wings so I can fly

Up and Down

Up and down
Round and round
Depressive thoughts
Driving me into the ground

No energy
No motivation
As my illness wreaks
It's devastation

No place to run
No where to hide
As I sit here
Contemplating suicide

But I don't want to die
I would prefer to live
It is just your loving care
That you need to give

Then you can help
Then you can support me
And hopefully one day
I will be back where I ought to be

Calling

I can not pretend
To be what I am not
You can interrogate me
You can put me on the spot
I keep no secrets from you
The truth is all I speak
And you should instinctively know
That once more I have become mentally weak
The pills and the potions
Don't seem to be doing their tricks
And I have become so terribly anxious
That it is making me physically sick
I had prayed that
This would never happen again to me
I thought I had learned
The Art of Escapology
But there is no fooling anyone
Least of all myself
I am at my wits end
And I'm calling out to you for help

Help! I Need Somebody

Help! I need somebody
Anyone will do
Anyone who can lift my mood
And stop me feeling blue

Help! I need somebody
Who will put meaning to my life
Anyone who can change my feelings
And stop this downward slide

Help! I need somebody
Anyone who can spare the time
To listen to my sad story
And stop this gradual decline

Help! I need somebody
Anyone could fit the bill
Anyone who can support me
And stop me becoming ill

Help! I need somebody
With their arms open wide
Ready to protect me
From that crazy world outside

MENTAL ILLNESS

Depression

How can I describe
The way I feel inside?
The endless thoughts that go round in my head
Convince me that I am emotionally dead
If you should search for my soul
You would just find a void or a great big hole
The very fabric that is me
Has been stripped away and now deserts me
I live in a world that promises nothing
So what is the point in bothering?
My life is like a jigsaw puzzle
Where all the pieces are in a muddle
I am in a state, I am in a mess
But there is no cure because there is no visible illness
Only God knows how much more
I can take of these pointless unrewarding chores
Sometimes the minutes feel like hours
But to change things will require some inner strength or
forgotten power
To get through the day can be an enormous task
And often poses questions that I dare not ask
Here I am with my internal strife
And if you look closely I have been condemned to life

Depressed

I have lost the ability to plan and look ahead
I can barely go to the shops to buy a loaf of bread
I often find it hard to do things as they are stipulated
And this leaves me feeling very frustrated
My self confidence is torn to shreds
I face each day with overwhelming dread
Fearing I will have no strength when it is needed
And unable to praise myself even when I have
succeeded
My progress is all the time being impeded
The things I thought I knew how to do have been
superseded
My life is being completely wasted
Being depressed is the bitterest pill I have ever tasted

Breaking Point

All my fantasies and dreams
Have been ripped apart at the seams
There has been another body blow
To my increasingly fragile ego
But I only have myself to blame for this situation
Because this circumstance is of my own creation
The things that are wrong are due to faults of mine
And the anomalies have been building up over time
Now everything seems to be out of joint
I have reached my breaking point

Shed a Tear

As I write this I shed a tear
It is trickling across my cheek
For once again I have let myself down
I have demonstrated that I am weak
Bang, Bang goes the pounding in my head
Slap, Slap my hands against my face
I am trying to knock some sense back in
From where it has escaped
Pull yourself together I say
Don't let things get out of hand
But I don't think I can do this anymore
I need to find the promised land
A place where I can shelter
To ride out this turbulent storm
That has been brewing up inside me
And now leaves me all forlorn
I am broken into a thousand shards
That need to be delicately re-stuck
But I don't know where to start
I feel like giving up

Nervous Breakdown

When you can hardly make a cup of coffee for yourself
Or cook a meal without needing help
If you can't even do the basic chores
Like doing the shopping or washing floors
Then it is time to recognise
That a 'nervous breakdown' is your demise
It is more than just being depressed
Your higher cognitive functions have been repressed
You can no longer care for number one
And something serious must be done
You will have to check into a clinic
Or you will be sectioned and forced to do it
They will care for you and keep you safe
Until you can recuperate
It may take a little while for things to improve
And reality may seem far removed
But with luck, medication and time
Your faculties will gradually come back on line
Soon you will be going home
And you can begin to cope again on your own
Eventually the day will come
When you find you are starting to have fun
The battle is over and the war is won
The rest of your life has just begun

Being Sectioned

They don't use straight jackets any more
But if they did they would have used one on me
For on that fateful day
I had become unhinged from reality
I had taken a load of drugs
And washed them down with alcohol
Trying to obliterate the world
Going against all logical protocol
I had also tried to slit my wrist
But it was a very lame attempt
I think it was a cry for help
A way to make the mental pain relent
I just wanted to change
The way I felt inside
I didn't care about the consequences
I didn't care that I might die
But my doctor set the alarm bells ringing
At the eleventh hour
And I was put on a 'section'
They took away all my power
I was taken to a place of safety
Where I could do no more damage
I was forced to stay in hospital
Where my illness could be managed
It was a very spartan place
And rather alien to me
But it saved me from myself
I could inflict no further injury
Looking back it is difficult to comprehend
Why I did these crazy things
But luckily I am still here to tell the tale
And prove that life really is worth living

Hospital

I understand now that I am ill
Because I feel that time is almost standing still
I count the minutes as they slowly pass
Questioning how long this depression will last
My only form of escape is to sleep
Then I am oblivious to these feelings that run so deep
I find it hard to relax or just sit in a chair
My legs are fidgety and that's driving me to despair
Often I will walk the length of the corridor
With no purpose because there is nowhere left to
explore
Up and down I pace all day long
Wondering if I have done something wrong
I have been hospitalised for my own safety
But it has happened in a way that is rather hasty
I know I should be here for my own protection
And I won't mount any form of insurrection
I am a danger to myself
Needing constant supervision and professional help
For now I am stuck in this loony bin
Fighting my battle against depression
And hoping one day I will win

Denial

Damn you all to kingdom come
Nothing is amiss, there is nothing wrong
So I don't need your help
Because I am not ill myself
You keep telling me I am acting strange
When in fact to me it is you who appears deranged
But I am strong and I can read your games
You are accusing me of being insane
I will play along for a while
To stop you saying I am in denial
I will utter all the things you want to hear
If that will get me out of here
The wool will be pulled over your eyes
And you won't know if I am telling lies
I am okay, I am alright
Now get out of my godforsaken sight

Walls

I am here of my own volition
But that doesn't stop it feeling like prison
I am confined by these four walls
I am incarcerated in this hospital
There is nothing to do except sit around
And this only makes my thoughts compound
Even though there are other people here
I still feel alone, I am close to tears
I miss the love of my family
There is no one who will console me
I am desperate to leave this place
But until I can learn how to correctly behave
I won't be going home
I will remain locked within these walls of stone

31

Sit

All I can do is sit and stare
Because my life is going no where
I am a poor lost soul
A square peg trying to fit into a round hole

All I can do is sit and wonder
Why my life has gone asunder
I am a tired spent force
A stream that has dried up at its source

All I can do is sit out my time
Hoping one day further down the line
My energy will be replenished
And the dark cloud hanging over me will vanish

All I can do is continue to sit
While I try to fathom out how I ended up like this
If only I had the answer to this question
Surely once and for all I could conquer my depression?

Suicidal

I think I am going to suffer a premature death
As I sit here trying to catch my breath
This will occur by my own hand
I just hope that you will understand
Recently nothing seems to be worthwhile
There has been nothing to make me raise a smile
I have been mulling things over in my head
I have decided you would be better off if I were dead
For my life has become empty and meaningless
Plus my affairs are a complete and utter mess
So let me end the pain today
Just let me slip away
Please don't cry
I want to die
Au revoir, so long, goodbye

Self Harm

My heart is beating fast
Adrenalin is pumping in my veins
I look down at the carpet
I can see the blood stains
Where is this red liquid from?
Is it coming from me?
I glance down at my arms
And it is plain to see
I have a knife in my hand
I have cut my wrist
I must have put the blade right in
And given it a twist
There is no way of stopping the blood
I need a piece of tape
Before the loss is fatal
And I exsanguinate
I am not sure if I am meant to die
Or inflict some tangible pain
But it looks like I have no choice
My life is ebbing all the same
Just in time my husband has appeared
He manages to stem the flow
I will have to visit the hospital
It is the logical place to go
Here they put some stitches in
My life has been spared
But I won't be going home yet
I must stay for some further care
They will monitor me closely
And make sure I don't relapse
I am not going to struggle
I am in a state of collapse
It has been a close call
But I am not ready to say goodbye
I will have to carry on
Or at least I'll have to try

Different

Sometimes I drink too much
Sometimes I take drugs I shouldn't touch
Sometimes I cut my arms which is obtuse
But these are all forms of self abuse
How do these acts help my situation?
For me they bring a temporary cessation
Of my immediate conscious experience
They serve to make me feel something different

No Choice

Bloody hell what have I done?
The wound I have inflicted is making me feel numb
Why do I do this to myself
When I only have to ask for help?
I am not sure I trust those around me
For all the things they say are persecutory
They tell me they will only go away
If I hurt myself without delay
They urge me down this route of pain
Reinforcing their message again and again
I try very hard to block out their voice
But in the end they insist I have no choice

The Crime

I must have committed a crime
Because I have lost my life's paradigm
I should, therefore, be punished
If I want my guilt to be diminished
What form will this punishment take?
Anything that will obviate
The pain that eats from inside out
The pain that makes me want to shout
And I am convinced I am to blame
For creating my depression once again

Self Mutilation

Pain, oh mental pain
It is driving me insane
There is a continuous ache
From which I can't escape
I need to find a distraction
Something that will give an immediate reaction
Maybe physical injury would be more bearable
Certainly the pain would be more understandable
I have found a blade with which to self harm
And I have outstretched my arm
The sharp steel cuts in deep
Although the blood that flows doesn't make me weep
My actions may not be circumspect
However they do have the desired effect
Briefly the tension and anxiety has eased
The hurt inside has been relieved
You may ask "Did you really mean to die?"
I give the answer "No" with a sigh
In fact the superficial cutting has helped me avoid
Actually committing suicide
And perhaps all I want is to highlight my situation
That is why I carry out self mutilation

Suicide

You can tell when I am depressed
And I am really feeling down
I tend to hunch my shoulders
And tip my head toward the ground
I say things like "I want to end it all"
And "I can't cope with any more of this"
I become very anxious
And overwhelmingly distressed
I only talk like this because
I can see no way out
There appears to be no option left
And this makes me want to scream and shout
The question is "Would I be able to do it?"
I am not sure that I can
It would require careful planning
For me to shorten my life span
At the moment I can't say what will happen
I am unable to decide
It would be a rather drastic measure
If I were to commit suicide
For now I will carry on
In the hope that I will find
Something worth living for
And a little peace of mind

Release

I want you to listen carefully to what I have to say
I'm not fooling about I am serious today
I have reached a point where I am in a trap
And to be honest I am feeling really crap
I loathe myself for creating this situation
But I can't take anymore I have reached saturation
I am engulfed by hatred for myself
Because I can't leave this drug up there on the shelf
I have consumed so much that I feel numb
And I am chastising myself for having succumbed
Have I taken a fatal dose? I hear you cry
I certainly hope so because I don't want to survive
I think the time has come for me to depart
And leave this world that has fallen apart
In death I will find my final release
I will be at one with God, I will be at peace

Nightmare

I don't know if you are aware
But I am living in a constant nightmare
Everything that can go wrong does
And there is no one to comfort me and give me love
I am locked in a never ending loop
And I am unable to jump through the right hoop
Although I put up noble resistance
I am left fighting for my own existence
I never seem to get on top
There is no way to make the nightmare stop

Crazy

The world is becoming rather dim and hazy
I am about to do something you may view as crazy
I am going to take an overdose of pills
Enough to end my life by making me fatally ill
The intention is for me to die
I can't explain or give a reason why
All I can say is that I feel bemused
As I sit here on a time bomb that can't be defused
It is ready to explode in my face
And I can't run away there is no escape
I can't work out how I ended up in this depressed
condition
Or why the prospect of death has become such a
tantalising proposition
If I am still with you as you are reading this
Then my mission has yet to be accomplished
Which leaves me time to apologise for all the anguish I
will cause
But you must understand I can't take anymore of these
mental wars

No More Rhymes

No more rhymes, no more poems
Because there is no where left to be going
I have reached a brick wall
I can't climb over it for I fear I will fall
There are so many problems troubling me
Each one on their own enough to defeat me
But added together they become insurmountable
Every day I face choices that are redoubtable
To day is the day that my agony will end
And I am writing to you to say thank you for being my
friend
I can see no way out except to take my own life
I will make it swift with this very sharp knife
I am sorry for the grief I will leave behind
Everyone has been so genuinely kind
Sorry, sorry, sorry I can say no more
But I must finally escape this place I deplore

As I Look

As I look around this empty space
I find a frown upon my face
Because I am an utter disgrace
But it is a situation from which I can't escape

As I look inside my empty mind
There is nothing there for me to find
And I feel like this all the time
Which ticks slowly by between the hourly chimes

As I look around this empty room
I find that I am totally consumed
By a feeling of impending doom
Just praying that I will be rescued soon

Unhappy

I am extremely unhappy
I am almost drowning in my tears
My worst nightmare has been realised
And there is no escape from all my fears
I am wallowing in self pity
And I am totally consumed
With these wretched thoughts
That only predict further doom
If there is a God in heaven
He appears to have forsaken me
I am struggling to keep my head above water
And to preserve my sanity
I am a complete failure
I have let everyone down
My face portrays my feelings
And I wear a permanent frown
I don't know where I will go from here
Or how I am going to survive
But if I decide to take my own life
Then do not be horrified

Where in the World

Where in the world am I supposed to go?
When there are people lurking in the shadows
Tell me please who I can trust?
And who will help me now that things are tough
I am suspicious of those who I meet
As I try to balance on my own two feet
One little push would send me falling
Into a depression so appalling
That there would be no escape
There would be no room to negotiate
As I teeter here on the brink
I have time to contemplate and think
Do I really want to die?
A question which still requires my reply

Alone

I am sitting here alone
Waiting for someone to come home
But I know they will never arrive
Because I have no one special in my life
My friends have all deserted me
And I have been abandoned by my family
I have driven them away
By the awful things that I say
But if they knew the pain I'm in
Then they would be more understanding
I am constantly wracked with grief
In a way that is beyond belief
And the horror with which I view the world outside
Cannot totally be described
I am tormented by my own self doubt
And this has made me shut everyone out
I am trapped inside my shell
In a place that resembles hell
I feel anxious, I feel lost
But I have sinned and now must pay the cost
Back in my room I continue to sit
I have told myself I must not quit
There must be a light at the end of the tunnel
Even if it is minuscule
I will have to focus it in my sight
And lock on to it until it becomes bright
Then one day maybe I won't be on my own
I won't be sitting here all alone

Warning Lights

I want you to know
That once again I have become ill
The warning lights are flashing
Even though I have taken the proper pills
I have started to withdraw
To hide away and avoid contact
I have lost interest in life
That is somewhat chilling but is the cold hard fact
What am I going to do?
Other than to isolate myself somewhere
I can't see how to stop sliding
Down the slippery slope to despair
My motivation has evaporated
I don't have the energy to keep pushing on
The driving force within me
Is running out fast and is almost gone
A lesion in my brain has been created
It has severed the centre for happiness
There is a total lack of emotion
And I am left with a sort of emptiness
It will take time for my mind to heal
To forge new pathways to replace what's missing
I know this is the cure to all my problems
But it is also what makes things ultimately depressing

Out of Control

God have mercy on my soul
For I am completely out of control
I can't see the wood for the trees
I am stranded in a world of make believe
Where do the boundaries of reality end?
Pray tell me just how far they extend
I am at the point where these two dimensions meet
And I am trying not to fall into the breach
I know I am teetering on the brink of insanity
Because I can't see things with any clarity
My behaviour has become somewhat erratic
My head is spinning as if on a piece of elastic
I can't channel my thoughts or concentrate
And my mind is looking for a way to escape
I feel my life has become totally bizarre
It will be easy for me to take that step too far

Normal

I want to feel normal
No longer depressed
I want to break free of this mindset
To which I have become obsessed
My thoughts keep spiralling downwards
One after the other
And I can't see any way
I will ever recover
The doctor has prescribed
Some tablets for me
And this should relieve the symptoms
And allow me back from obscurity
But whether they work or not
Only time will tell
Until then I will continue
In this living hell

I have been here before though
And somewhere deep inside
I know that I will get better
And the pain will subside
I cling to the hope
That I will eventually be
Feeling back to normal
And being the real me

Being Ill

I know I have been very ill
Several times in the past
Each occurrence is distressing
And I pray it will be the last
No matter how I try to protect myself
Or the protests that I make
Depression is in grained in me
And it is very difficult to shake
But the periods of being well
Are lengthening all the time
The mountains that lead to recovery
Are not as difficult to climb
I can also identify
The subtle changes in my thinking
Hopefully before I get so low
That I can't stop my ship from sinking
I never want to be hospitalised again
I never want to have suicidal thoughts
Because it is really hideous
Being that completely overwrought
I live my life one day at a time
I don't look too far into the future
And I continue to nurse this open wound
That may still need some sort of suture

Doldrums

My mind is unbalanced
I am feeling detached from reality
I don't know which way to turn
There is no end to my misery
I want to scream out loud
So everyone can hear
That I am in the doldrums
From which there is no way out I fear
I am waiting for the winds of change
To fill my flaccid sails
And give my ship that is becalmed
A new direction where hope can prevail
But I have to help the mist disperse
I can't stand idly by
I know I must put some effort in
If the situation is to be rectified
I must tap into my inner strength
My hidden energy reservoir
That has kept me going
And has allowed me to come this far
Hesitantly I move forward then
Not knowing what lies in my path
Praying that each day in the doldrums
Will turn out to be my last

Swings and Roundabouts

As a child I loved to swing free
On a rope tied to the apple tree
Backwards and forwards reaching high
In a way that would almost death defy

As a child I loved to spin out
On an old and rusty roundabout
Round and round until I was dizzy
In a way that would almost make me queasy

As a child I didn't have a care
Life was one continual fun fair
Up and down on the carousel
In a way that never ceased to thrill

As an adult this has all gone
Responsibilities have come along
Now its swings and roundabouts in my head
Making a world of misery instead

Sometimes I wish I were a child once more
Life was simple then and not a chore
I wish that someone would look after me
And push me again on that swing in the apple tree

The Trenches

I am entrenched in a depressive land
The enemy is only a stone's throw away
I must attack, well that's the plan
But many obstacles stand in my way

My feet are rooted to the spot
The mud is sucking me back
I can't seem to push myself over the top
The energy required I sorely lack

You can point a gun at my head
To try to make me comply
I can only wish I were home in bed
For I am not ready yet to die

Can't we call a truce?
Can't you let me live again?
But sometimes I think 'What's the use'
There will always be this mental pain

I continue to brawl with this depression so evil
In the hope that I will find some extra strength
To eventually defeat my devil
I am prepared to go to any lengths

You see I will never completely give up
For I believe I can still win the war
One day reinforcements will come with a bit of luck
And then I can finally settle the score

Declining Mood

My mood has started to decline
It has begun to slip away
The foundations of my world
Are starting to decay
I am being pulled down
And I am already half submerged
But I am trying desperately
To keep my systems purged
As depression tries to drag me
And once more suck me under
I ask myself the question
Why has my life gone asunder?
But there is nothing
You can put your finger on
That would easily explain
Why I have reached my Armageddon
Is it a battle I can win?
Is it a war to end all wars?
I don't know but I continue to fight
In the hope I will one day be the victor

Self Destruct

As I spill my heart out onto this page
The words become deeply engraved
For I am trying to express
This lonely feeling, this emptiness
I can't think what I am supposed to do
So I just sit here and stew
Of course this only makes matters worse
I have been struck down by depression's curse
Funnily enough I don't feel like crying
Although there is no denying
That I am very down in the mouth
I just don't have the energy to let it all out

This house is somewhere I should feel secure
But its creature comforts have no allure
The walls act as my prison cell
Encasing me in a living hell
Do you see where I am coming from?
A place of pain and where the suffering is long
I tell myself my power must not be relinquished
I must not let my internal flame be extinguished
By adhering to the rules of good conduct
I will not allow myself to self destruct

Why?

Why do I hate myself so much?
Why do I keep beating myself up?
Why do I crumple when things get tough?
Why don't I have any backbone as such?

Why do I have to lean on others as an emotional
crutch?
Why is it so hard to find anyone I can trust?
Why can't I stop this anxiety that comes with such a
rush?
Why do I constantly need help? Why is that a must?

I don't have the answers to these questions
And there has never been any suggestion
That there is an adequate way of expression
Except to say I am suffering from "Depression"

The Return

Today I skived off work
I couldn't face what needed to be done
So I decided to call in sick
Until my imaginary pain had gone
But am I in fact mentally ill?
Has my depression returned?
Certainly I don't feel myself
And maybe there should be cause for concern
I lack energy and motivation
A feeling of apathy pervades
My thoughts are stuck in a never ending loop
And their contents are retrograde
Now must be the time for me
To practise what I preach
I must bring my coping strategies into effect
While they are still within my reach
I understand that I must persevere
I mustn't give up on myself
And if I can't manage on my own
Then I can always ask for help

Cease to Exist

Thoughts in my head of depression are being repeated
I question how my life will ever be completed
The same old nagging doubts as before
And the feeling that I can't cope anymore
In fact I have given up on myself
I don't think anyone else can really help
This is a personal vendetta fraught with danger
A serious disease, but not something that's contagious
I wish others could say they truly understand
But if they've never been "in depression" I don't see
how they ever can
My world is the worst place you can possibly picture
I am cast adrift on the sea without a safety fixture
Bobbing up and down I try to gulp in air now and then
Before being dragged down into this watery dungeon
I feel I am drowning I am finding it difficult to breathe
There is a great pressure in my chest making me want
to heave
My head is spinning wildly
And I see things very vividly
Body and mind are disconnected
Even though I try to keep it all in perspective
I take the medication as prescribed
It is that alone that keeps me alive
I would dearly love to click my fingers
And heal the part of my brain that's injured
Still I accept that there is no miracle cure
But that doesn't stop me clutching at straws
I hope one day the straw won't slip through my grip
Because if that doesn't happen then I may cease to
exist

Broken Brain

Snap, Snap
Something broke in my brain
Crack, Crack
My mind can't take the strain
The grey matter in my head has lost its fight
Right in the middle of the night
Just when somnolence should send me fast asleep
All I want to do is to cry and weep
Back and forth in the room I pace
Searching for someway out of this isolated place
In fact I sway to and fro
Clutching the furniture as I go
Hell hath no fury like the pain I'm in
Maybe I should end it now and stop the suffering
I know that is crazy talk
As I continue to walk
Praying, hoping, trusting the life I had on a plate
Will be returned to me at some later date

What Will Tomorrow Bring?

What will tomorrow bring?
Will I be able to cope with everything?
I am not sure I will survive
For there are many troubles in my life
The root of my problem is
The constant combat I have with mental illness
And no matter how hard I endeavour
To pull myself together
I am often overwhelmed
Feeling that I am dragged into another realm
I am on the outside looking in

A voyeur of the world and the tragedy therein
There is no sense that I belong
I am not in tune with anyone else's song
So I have to take myself out of the equation
To remove myself from general circulation
Until my brain has healed and re-adjusted
And my intuition can once more be trusted

Wish

As I wend my way to bed I make a wish
That tomorrow won't turn out to be the same as this
Because I've been feeling really 'bad'
I've been living in the worst nightmare I've ever had
All my plans have been curtailed
My life has gone completely off the rails
I have no energy, no drive
There is nothing to make me want to be alive
I get no pleasure from my day
All my emotion has slowly ebbed away
This means I have lost all purpose
Making me feel utterly worthless
So as I make this one small wish
I hope that when I wake my problems will have
vanished

Losing my Sanity

Today I cannot focus
I'm all over the place
My mind's all jumbled up
It's a confused and turbulent space
I want to do something constructive
I want to change the way I think
But my brain can't get its act together
There is a missing link
Perhaps if I go to sleep
I will wake up refreshed
And all my thoughts will be more ordered
No longer in a mess
Tomorrow may be different
And everything will click
Consciousness is a strange state
No one really knows what makes us tick
So if I lose my sanity
What does this really mean?
There is nothing you can put your finger on
It is something quite unseen
No one can explain it
They don't know where to start
It comes from deep within you
It's connected to the heart
If I go completely bonkers
You shouldn't really worry
One day I'll come right back to you
But it may not be in a hurry
Time is such a healer
Time helps the soul to mend
There is just one thing to remember
That I'll still be here in the end

Schizophrenia

Do you understand
What schizophrenia is like?
It is not having a split personality
That is purely hype
What it feels like is
Almost the same as being a child
The here and now is accentuated
The world becomes excessively wild
Your brain has too much dopamine
It can't make the right neurones connect
Reality becomes slightly warped
And it becomes difficult to recollect
Occasionally you might do something odd
Like laughing when a person dies
Your emotions are all heightened
They are intensified
You shouldn't worry about violence
Most schizophrenics won't hurt
They may be unpredictable
But there are drugs on hand that work
I hope this has enlightened you
Because there are many sufferers of this condition
People who need our help
And a little recognition

Worst Enemy

Sometimes I fear for my safety
Because I am my own worst enemy
I do things that are unpredictable
That only go to show I am unstable
Even when my life is going well
I still put myself in situations from hell
Almost like a game or initiative test
To see if I have what it takes to come out best
This can be very frightening
Because what if I fail to win
That is when you send me
To see the doctor of psychiatry
He drugs me up to make me behave
He stops me from rattling my cage
But I am very mischievous
The things I do are very devious
And while I continue to have a lark
Most of the time I keep you in the dark

Paranoia

What have I done to deserve this?
I thought I was at the helm of a steady ship
What was the thing that tipped the balance?
So that I am permanently in abeyance
I feel spaced out, a little detached
I'm sure a plot against me is being hatched
Who is involved I'm not quite sure
It may even include the stupid doctors
For they are playing silly games with me
Locking me up and throwing away the key
They twist my words to make them incriminate
And refuse to discharge me with any haste

I am clear in my mind that I am not ill
But they continue to force down the poisonous pills
To try to leave would be futile
For they are watching all the while
And they are so patronising
Which they never show any intent of disguising
Do you think that I am paranoid?
Or am I justified in being annoyed?

Delusions

Please don't give me that look so austere
I don't want you to think I am insincere
You should accept me as I first appear
Because to me my thoughts are very clear

Please don't give me that look of despise
What I am telling you is not a pack of lies
It is not fabricated or contrived
And I don't have any demons to be exorcised

Please don't give me that look of condemnation
I am not your delusional poor relation
What I am experiencing is real not a hallucination
If you want I can show you my stamp of authentication

Please don't give me that look of consternation
Maybe my mind does need to be straightened
Perhaps what is happening is strange on reflection
I think after all I do require your protection

Please tell me if this is the case
It seems I may have been living my life in a daze
And I may need your help without delay
Because if I am imagining things I must be half crazed

Tormenters

I seek to draw attention to myself
Because deep down I know that I need help
I don't mind if it is by a negative act
All I want to do is to attract
I receive weird messages inside my head
From tormenters who suggest I would be better off
dead
Then you wouldn't have to suffer my odd behaviour
And you could be relieved from your role as my saviour
Gone would be the emotional outbursts
That inflict such pain and only serve to hurt
You wouldn't have to see me waste away
Or witness my decline into a complete zombie
For that is what I am sure I will become
And you must admit it doesn't sound like fun
I say all this to make you aware
That things have gone beyond your duty of care
And for now as I take my leave
I fear one day my tormenters will be appeased

Voices

Do you hear voices?
Or imagine things that aren't really there?
It can be very frightening
And give you a nasty scare
For me they only come
When I am seriously depressed
They are a symptom of my illness
And occur when I am under undue stress
To begin with I thought the voices were real
Not a figment of my imagination
I was unable to detach myself
Or view them with any rationalisation
Now I understand what is happening
My mind is playing silly tricks
I don't pay them so much attention
I know they are only there because I am sick
Luckily there is medication I can have
That keeps the callers at bay
It stops them taking over
And I don't let them spoil my day
But if you are suffering
With demons of your own
Tell them to bugger off
And that your house is not their home!

Manic Depression

My mood is unstable
It cycles up and down
I seem to ricochet back and forth
And often wear a puzzled frown
When times are good
I can put the world to right
Flying up above the clouds
Just like a soaring kite
But hang on a minute
Didn't I say have a type of depression?
I sometimes dive to great depths
That is the nature of my condition
I long for the day
When I am in the middle
My mind will be more balanced
And I will have solved life's riddle
Here in my world
I see things in black and white
Both sides of the coin are visible
And I often feel contrite
Because I think I should be in control
I should be able to stop these swings
But this proves to be impossible
I am stuck with my extreme feelings
When I go to bed at night
I try to imagine my future running smoothly
However on waking up I find
There is nothing with which to soothe me
If you can associate
With everything I've said
You will recognise my dilemma
And that I am another one of the cursed

My Life's Score

I have been to hell and back
Struck down again by a savage depressive attack
I had prayed this wouldn't happen anymore
Because I thought I had learned how to read my life's
score
That, however, was not the case
And I guess it is a problem I will always have to face
I know the drugs I take are vital
But still my mood swings continue to cycle
I haven't given up though my fight goes on
The period of the cycles is becoming ever more
prolonged
This means I can take pleasure in being with my family
Caring for them and enjoying their company
I don't set my targets unrealistically high
Despite the fact that at times I feel I could fly
At the end of the day I have to be satisfied with my lot
And hope that I never completely lose the plot

Being Manic

I can't stop my brain from churning
It is driving me to distraction
I don't want to sleep because
Everything has so much attraction
I try to switch it off
What more can I do
Maybe I should learn to meditate
And that would see me through
But on the other hand
I am having lots of fun
And who would want to change?
When there is so much to be done
I feel that the sky's the limit
Nothing is out of my reach
Pardon me for being rude
But I don't mean to preach
I try to stay in control
And on top of the situation
Because this is mania
And it can be a dangerous affliction

Dark Day/Bright Day

What makes a dark day even darker?
What makes a bright day even sparklier?
I can't put my finger on it
If I knew that I would have to be a fountain of all
knowledge
Sometimes when the sun is shining outside
I am muddled and churned up on the inside
And yet other days pass like a beautiful dream
So why should my life be made up of these extremes?
I think it may be related to being ill
And in recognising this I have to swallow that bitter pill
You may find it hard to comprehend that I have no
control
Especially when my life is great and my virtues are
extolled
But when the good times are over
You will see I am not lying in a bed of clover
Rather I am lost within myself
Unable to function like everyone else
I start each day with fear and trepidation
Not knowing whether there will be depression or
elation
The future then holds much uncertainty
And being a manic depressive means my world is full
of disparity

Mood Swings

I can't help feeling blue
There is nothing I can do
I have an illness where my mood swings
But it is hard to accept I have no control of these things
There is an imbalance of brain chemicals
And to change that is almost impossible
So I have to take the medicine prescribed
To stop my life going completely awry
But I don't mean to moan
For the seeds of hope have been sown
I will make the most of the highs
Always remembering I can touch the sky
While being aware that there will be downs
Where I feel trapped underground
It is a very painful condition
But experience has given me better ammunition
To shoot away what holds me back
So that for a time I can stave off these dreadful attacks

On A High

When I am on a high
I can be quite flamboyant
I spend lots of money
For shear enjoyment
I start to plan
Weird and wonderful things to do
Despite the fact they are impossible
And nothing I say rings true
A false sense of confidence
Oozes from every pore
You wouldn't be able to stop me
Even with a twelve bore
My thoughts race
At a million miles an hour
I can't slow them down
And anyway I don't have the will power
My mind buzzes
Twenty four seven
I am busy all the time
I am in seventh heaven
Often I shout instructions
To those in my vicinity
So you had better watch out
For I don't suffer fools gladly
Energy, energy, energy
I am full of it
But there is one major drawback
I just don't know when to quit

MENTAL ILLNESS
RELATED PROBLEMS

Hiding

I hide away in my bedroom
With the curtains drawn
Cowering beneath the sheets
Trying to keep warm
I don't want to venture out
I don't want to start the day
There is nothing that appeals
And the chores can be delayed
I pull up my duvet
Firmly around my face
Glimpsing myself in the mirror
Oh what a terrible disgrace
I look like I have been
Pulled through a hedge backwards
I am a complete and utter mess
The world and I are in total discord
I don't have a job
I don't have any money
My life holds nothing for me
It is not a land of milk and honey
I know that hiding
Only puts off the inevitable
That somehow, sometime
I must face up to this life that's cruel
But how to break free
From the clutches of depression
When the negative thinking trap I'm in
Has become a self perpetuating obsession
Hang on in and give it time

Give it time you repeatedly say
The answer will elucidate itself
It will be unveiled to you some day
I am sure this is sound advice
But at the present it gives me no relief
So I continue to hide under the covers
Searching for my self belief

Panic

I have reached a dead end
And there is no way of going back
The walls are closing in
I am having a panic attack
My heart rate is going up
I think that I will die
My anxiety level is rising
Sending my blood pressure sky high
Everything is so intense
I am finding it difficult to breathe
I want to run away
But I don't know which way to leave
I collapse on the floor
In a crumpled mess
And strangers gather round
To add to my distress
But in minutes it is over
I begin to calm down
I start to pull myself together
And get up from on the ground
I slowly pick up my things
And head toward the exit
I know the attack is finished
And I am going to make it
When I question myself later
As to why this should happen to me
All I can say is that
"I'm a failure and it is my destiny"

Fill the Time

I have been up since dawn
Even though I continue to yawn
Sleep is what I crave but it eludes me
Because my brain is trying to confuse me
It is fixated on one thing
How do I get from morning to evening?
I don't know how to fill the time
And I have lost my life's paradigm
I am already agitated
For the day appears to be elongated
The hours stretch out before me
There is nothing to break the monotony
I could just sit here all day
And let the time tick slowly away
But there must be more to life than this
Something has gone seriously amiss
Where do I go? Who do I see?
Who will re-educate me?
If I could understand where I went wrong
I could learn how to be strong
Then this illness could be sent into remission
There would be a chance to end my depression

What If?

What if I had never been ill?
What if I didn't have to take these wretched pills?
Sometimes I dwell on the situation
For I would dearly love to stop the medication
But the risks are so great
It is not something I should contemplate
In fact I should be happy with the status quo
I shouldn't want to rock the boat
However it doesn't stop me asking
What if there was a treatment that was long lasting?
Then I could throw the tablets in the bin
And it wouldn't be seen as a mortal sin
At some point I'm sure this will be the case
And all my antidepressants can be laid to waste

Olanzapine

Olanzapine is the drug I choose
To stop me feeling so confused
It quashes my anxiety
And tempers my sobriety
The racing thoughts are halted in their tracks
And the weird voices cease with their attacks
I even find my mood is more stable
So you see this medicine is very valuable
But "Where's the catch?" I hear you exclaim
Well it is the problem of excessive weight gain
That in turn lays me open to diabetes
And I have to give up all those tempting sweeties
It is cruel that it should work this way
Because since olanzapine was added to my armoury
I have become increasingly mentally well
And I don't want to do anything that breaks the spell

Side Effects

I fear I have become
Merely an automaton
Controlled by a computer program
That dictates just who I am
The drugs prescribed for my depression
Stifle me and put me in this position
Although in many ways they are beneficial
The change in my personality is more than superficial
The medication also saps my energy
And makes me feel a little drowsy
Then it becomes hard to decide
Who I really am inside
But despite these unwanted side-effects
I won't forget to take my tablets
Because without them I don't function at all
They stop me stepping in any pitfalls
And at the end of the day I choose
To take the medicine and accept the lesser of two evils

Memory

My illness has affected my memory
It is not as reliable as it used to be
I tend to repeat myself more than once
In a way that causes me to appear a dunce
Only my memory of things just past
Is altered and makes me feel aghast
Whereas my thoughts of times long gone
Remain set in tablets of stone
I know that for my memory to improve
I need to exercise it and put it to good use
Then the neural pathways will of course
Be strengthened and reinforced

Get a Grip

Do I have a virus?
Or is this self inflicted pain?
I can't tell the difference
The symptoms are the same
I have stopped taking my medication
The pills are in the bin
Because I am fed up with
The lethargy they bring
My muscles ache
And my joints are stiff
My head is spinning
I have come adrift
All those things I said
About helping myself to stay strong
Have flown out the window
The good intentions have all gone
I pick myself up
And dress myself down
I must force a smile
As I try to turn it around
Positive thinking must win through
I will have to make a stand
And listen to my own good advice
That may allow me to once more take command
With a bit of luck and good fortune
I will overcome this blip
The only way to achieve this
Is to take life firmly in my grip

I Must Change

My vision is clouded by my tears
As I am having to face up to all my fears
I can't run away and hide
Now is the time to look things in the eye
I may not like what I see
But that will not deter me
I need to clarify the situation
And then find a source of inspiration
A different way of life must be found
Or I'll end up six feet under ground
I have put on a vast amount of weight
So I must be more active and not vegetate
I must stop spending money or being lavish
Forking out just because it has become a habit
I must give more of myself to my family
I will have to find that inner capacity
I must learn to love who I am
I must change
I know I can

A Deep Breath

Take a deep breath in
Count to ten
Try to relax
And the world will cease to spin
I am reeling with
The effects of drug withdrawal
I have taken a monumental step
I only hope that I don't slip and fall
But this is a positive move
With me in control
I am, am I not
The one looking to mend their soul?

I am searching for the sparkle
That used to be so bright
It enabled me and gave me strength
It illuminated a path of pure delight
I will get back the drive
That allowed me to achieve so much
I no longer need these drugs
As an emotional crutch
Say a prayer for me
That I have made the correct move
Nothing ventured nothing gained
I still have a point to prove!

Lost Identity

I feel like I am just another number
Being shipped from pillar to post
No one takes me seriously
And that's what hurts the most
Can't you see that I require help?
From a kind and caring person
Who will nurse me back to health
Making sure my illness doesn't worsen
I need someone to take me under their wing
And protect me from the world outside
To give me a chance to preen my feathers
So that once more I can fly
I am searching for a mentor
Who will show I have true abilities
A friend who will give me my life back
And confirm my lost identity

Failure

If I fail to achieve
If I don't reach my goals
Am I a worthless person?
Is this a reflection on my soul?
Do I chastise myself
Every time something goes wrong?
Do I dish out punishment?
Or is this a little too strong?
In fact I should look closely
And analyse the situation
For all may not be lost
I should give myself some congratulations
Even though this time I didn't get there
Many lessons have been learned
Things aren't always handed out on a plate
Sometimes they have to be earned
Tomorrow is another day
I have the chance to try once more
And even if ultimately I don't succeed
I should still give myself a round of applause

Insecurity

I feel helpless and insecure
Like a child on their first day at school
Trying to keep within the boundaries
While not knowing all the rules

I feel worried and frightened
That if I put one foot out of place
A ton of bricks will be dropped on me
Or that I will fall flat on my face

I feel that I am living on a knife edge
One that is very sharp
Fearful that I will hurt myself
If I move too fast

I feel that I am being watched
The ground is giving way from beneath my feet
My credibility is being questioned
Making me feel weak

I feel that I lack power
I always give in and capitulate
I am so insecure
That I can't retaliate

Self Confidence

I lack self confidence
I shy away from responsibility
This is because I have no self belief
And judge myself too critically
I don't feel I am worthy
Of other people's faith
I don't think I am capable
And their expectations are too great
What can I do
To change this situation?
I will have to challenge myself
And do some experimentation
That way I can prove
One way or the other
Whether I am useless
Or really rather clever
I know that self confidence
Doesn't develop overnight
But if can banish these seeds of doubt
Then I can tip the balance right
One day I would like
To turn to you and say
I am feeling confident
And everything's going to be okay

No Self Belief

I have no self belief
It has been whittled away
By the adverse events
That seem to happen every day

I have no self confidence
When I do something it always goes wrong
So I have given up trying
I just sit here feeling that I don't belong

I have no self esteem
I have lost my faith
I am so traumatised
This depression has left me subjugate

Anxious

I am anxious and apprehensive
About what lies ahead
The unknown cannot be planned for
Despite all those books I've read
I worry all the time
That I won't be able to cope
For if there is no way to be prepared
Then all I can do is sit and mope
I would like to be more carefree
And let my life unfold naturally
But I don't possess this skill
I say quite ashamedly
I need someone to be a teacher
To show me how to be more relaxed
I want them to guide me
And lead me down the right track
I pray the day will come
When I can manage on my own
And I won't be in hospital anymore
I will be back in the sanctuary of my home

Anxiety

I am about to sit an exam
My hands are clammy with sweat
I have butterflies in my stomach
And I feel as though I am about to wretch
But in a few short hours it will be all over
And the anxiety will have disappeared
With a bit of luck I have passed
And I will be able to lay to rest all my fears
This illustrates a common circumstance
Where anxiety is to be expected
But what if you felt like this all the time
How would your life be affected?
When depression pulls me under
This is one of the symptoms I am up against
There is no apparent reason for feeling this way
I can't explain why I am so tense
Except to say that I dread being alive
I don't know how to structure my day
I don't think I will be able to cope
With whatever life chooses to throw my way`
This constant turmoil is very destructive
My confidence is completely undermined
It is a situation that can only be resolved
By me finding an inner strength of some kind

Inadequacy

I am starting to crumble at the edges
I need propping up with sturdy wedges
My very soul is decaying
And I have given up on praying
For if there really is a God
He appears to have given me the shove
How could he allow me to suffer so?
Wouldn't he have tried to soften the blow?
Once again I find myself in a depressed state
And there is no way to alleviate
All the feelings of inadequacy
That go round and round inside of me
I fear I can't be saved from a lingering death
Of this I become more certain with every single breath
But can't I survive a little longer?
Isn't there a piece of me that's stronger?
That clutches to life however tenuously
And keeps me fighting no matter how hard that may be
My spirit may have waned into a mere glow
But that is enough to re-ignite an inferno
And when the moment is right
I will be ready to step forward into the light

Not Good Enough

I am just not good enough
For anyone to want to give me love
I let people down and I am unreliable
In a crisis I would be useless that's undeniable
I lie and cheat to get my own way
That is the pattern day after day
I will lead you up the garden path
While still keeping you very much in the dark
Hiding from you my real self
The one who is desperately in need of help
Outwardly I may seem as tough as old boots
But the devil and I are in cahoots
So in fact I am weak of mind
And I am hoping you could help me find
That zest for life which has disappeared
And happiness even if it has to be engineered

Problems

Today the sun is shining
And all the flowers are in full bloom
But I don't feel happy
My thoughts are filled with gloom
I can't sort out my problems
I have tried but I have failed
And all my good intentions
Have been completely derailed
I had hoped that by now
I would have made some sort of progress
But I am my own worst enemy
That much I must confess
When I feel this way
I want to relinquish all responsibility
I don't want to be relied upon
I have lost confidence in me
Where do I go from here?
Is the next question to be asked
I will have to put on a brave face
Or simply wear a mask
That way I can minimise
The effect I have on others
However my problems won't have disappeared
They will just remain under cover
I don't know what the future holds
And whether I will find my life's solution
But I know I should be punished
There must be some kind of retribution

Drug Addict

I have a confession to make
That may make you want to cry
I have become a drug addict
And I don't know the reason why
I am completely hooked
That much I know for certain
It has changed my life
And turned me into a different person
I spend a lot of time and money
Looking for the next fix
I have become very devious
And use lots of clever tricks
You can't begin to understand
The total relief I feel
When the next batch of drug
Is finally revealed
I would like to give it up
But I don't know where to start
I mean that sincerely
From the bottom of my heart
The most drastic way to cure me
Would be to lock me in a padded cell
And then everyone could watch me
As I slowly go through hell
I have tried cutting down
But then I begin to cheat
Because the craving is so great
And the drug is my 'little treat'
I don't know how to turn things around
Or where to find help
But I am no longer in denial
I am being honest with myself
If you think you can help me
Please let me know
Because I have reached a crisis point
And I don't know which way to go

Thin Ice

The mind is a fickle thing
It can be duped into believing
That it requires props and supports
To keep it operating in the way it ought
Mine thinks it needs this special drug
That I drink each day in one straight slug
It is not illegal or against the law
And it can be bought from any chemist's store
Each day I start with good intentions
Not to take this chemical I mention
But at some point I always acquiesce
Because I become so terribly distressed
I don't think I have an actual addiction
It is just a habit this affliction
I now feel sorry for those trying to give up smoking
It is difficult to stop, I am not joking
I pray each night when I go to bed
That tomorrow I will be able to turn things on their head
I also pray I don't take an overdose
Leaving me permanently comatose
And you should not condone this way of life
For I am sure I am skating on thin ice

Temptation

I cannot resist temptation
When it is placed in front of me
I don't understand the meaning of "No Thank You"
It is not part of my vocabulary
I have no self control
And show no inner discipline
I am easily lured
Into doing the wrong thing
I know quite well
That if something appears too good to be true
Then it probably is just that
And I mustn't get confused
All too often I am tempted
I can't stick to the righteous path
And I have to suffer the consequences
Or any terrible aftermath

Set Me Free

I am very worried about my general health
And I don't mean the state of my inner self
I think that physically I am doing damage
By continuously taking more drugs than I can actually
manage
I am sure it is eating my insides away
Because I keep taking it day after day
But how do I bring an end to this dependency?
Which is the button I must press to release me?
I would like to purge my system of these chemicals
And be rid of my problem by some small miracle
But I am weak and I can't keep the promises I make
It is too easy to continue with this terrible mistake
I don't know what the cure will ultimately be
Perhaps you could wave your magic wand and set me
free

Giving Up

Some day I will have to make a resolution
That I am going to stop taking this drug solution
I know this will be the correct decision
And I can predict the effects with some precision
I will get withdrawal symptoms at the start
And the craving will try to tear me apart
But I will reap the benefit in the end
Because my mind and body will start to mend
This will be one of the biggest steps I have ever taken
And you must think I am God forsaken
But please keep your fingers crossed for me
And hope in time I will succeed

Saviour

I have a plan for stopping my addiction
It is not another story or a work of fiction
I am going to stay at my parent's house
I am going to give myself a well deserved time out
I will relieve myself of responsibility
To become a child again with someone caring for me
My parents will restrain me and lock all the doors
And I won't have access to these drugs any more
Hopefully this will break the pattern of behaviour
And this action will turn out to be my saviour
I know it won't be easy and I am mentally prepared
But I know the problem will be halved when it is shared

You Don't Understand

You don't understand me
All you want to do is reprimand me
You would like to command me
To stop this behaviour that makes such demands of
me

Why do I follow this path so strange?
Is it possibly that I am deranged?
But I would truly like to change
And return to whence I came

Then I could start with a clean slate
And I wouldn't make the same mistakes
That only serve to complicate
And raise barriers between us that are difficult to
negotiate

So I hold out my hand to you
Hoping you will pull me through
Desperate to begin my life anew
A life I long to share with you

My Life

I remain emotionally scarred
By my constant battle with mental illness
I don't think I will ever fully recover
And get back to my original prowess
I used to be a confident person
Very sure of myself
I never needed guidance
I never needed anyone's help
Now I find that
I am constantly looking for reassurance
I doubt my own capabilities
And I question my endurance
But I must count my blessings
My husband has stood by me through thick and thin
Even when I have tested his patience
He has never thought of leaving
I have tried to protect my children
From my variable mood
Their upbringing has been as normal as possible
Despite my depressive interludes
In some ways I have been lucky
Not to have remained a nervous wreck
I still function reasonably well
My life is better than you might expect

Mistake

My thoughts are going round and round
Everyone is against me or so I've found
I have done something terribly wrong
And to put it right I'll need to be strong
I know that I am at fault
But I need the matter to be drawn to a halt
I can't change what I did
If I could I would have rectified it
I have made this dreadful mistake
I know the consequences, I know what is at stake
However I don't think I am entirely to blame
Because you should realise I am totally insane

Fear

When I told you I had been depressed
I could feel your fear
You took a noticeable step back
And put your hands over your ears
For you didn't like
What I had to say
You didn't want to listen
You began to shy away
It was clear that the stigma
Surrounding being mentally unwell
Had been indoctrinated in you
Your ignorance would be hard to dispel
But I am going to pin you down
And set the record straight
You must be enlightened
Before it is too late
Being mentally ill doesn't mean
Your brain has been removed
And there are many treatments
To make the situation improve

The sufferer needs help and support
Like with any other disease
They still need love and care
If they are to recover fully
You shouldn't be frightened
About saying the wrong thing
Just by being there to talk to
You will already be helping
So reach out your hand
And find the true person within
Be someone who has mental health awareness
Make a difference to those who are suffering

Discrimination

I am angry today
Because there has been discrimination
I may lose my job
As a result of my depression
I have missed time off work
That I cannot deny
But at no stage was the intention
To make the records falsified
I have not acted fraudulently
I have done everything in good faith
Nobody has suggested till now
That the figures don't equate
I want to set the record straight
And be given another chance
To prove to everybody
I am not leading them a merry dance
I apologise for what has happened
But there is no going back
This problem has only arisen
Because I have suffered another depressive attack

Targets

I am at my wits end
Not knowing what to do
I am afraid for myself
And that I have bitten off more than I can chew
Are my goals unrealistic?
Are they more than I can achieve?
Are my targets ridiculous?
Am I really that naïve?
This is the root of my problems
Always wanting to be the best
Striving for that pinnacle
And putting myself to the test
There is no easy answer
Even though I can see where I am going wrong
I still can't break the habits of a lifetime
Or escape this rut I have been in for so long
I want then for you to understand
Why I chastise myself so
But pray that one day I will change
And stop hiding from my own shadow

Precarious Situation

I have dug myself
Into a hole
But the events that have lead me here
Are beyond my control
I didn't choose
To be in this position
It is part and parcel
Of my depressive condition
My dreams have been shattered
I only wanted to live a normal life
But to make matters worse
Others have decided to stick in the knife

I walk a tight rope
Between being ill and being well
I am in a precarious situation
And I fear that no one would catch me if I fell
I try very hard
To operate within the boundaries set
But this is not always possible
Because I can't predict when depression will strike next
I hope that someone out there
Will have the sense to realise
That I never asked to be like this
And I should not be penalised

The Attack

You can make my life hell
You can send me to kingdom come
Push me as hard as you like
But I will not succumb
If you try to pull the carpet
From beneath my feet
You will not succeed
Because I am not someone who is weak
You cannot suppress me
Or break my indomitable spirit
The weight that you bring to bear
Will not make me submit
I have a strength of character
That puts you to shame
Making all your insidious remarks
Appear completely inane
I will not be stopped
There will be no holding me back
So you might just as well
Call off the attack

Conspiracy

All I want to do
Is hide away and burst into tears
Because my world is disintegrating
Everything is falling down around my ears
I thought that my life
Was on an even keel
But quite suddenly I have lost
Those feelings that were so surreal
I have been jolted
Back into reality
And it appears that
There really are people out to get me
They are determined
To show I have done wrong
And now I realise
They have been conspiring against me all along
I know in my heart
That I am innocent of the allegations
But it is hard to believe
There can't be some sort of reconciliation
Whatever happens next
My conscience is clear
I know I have nothing to feel guilty about
Therefore I have nothing left to fear

Lie Down and Die

I think I might as well lie down and die
Let me tell you the reason why
The life I live has been undermined
It is caving in and I can't press rewind
There are perpetrators as we speak
Whose sole purpose is to attack me when I am weak
They believe that I am guilty
Before seeing the evidence that shows I acted
innocently
These people are deliberately trying to trip me up
And are determined to make me come unstuck
I wish that they would go away
Because they are making my life a misery
I am looking for a way out
Before the pain is so great I have to shout

Sacrifice

I feel like giving up
I feel I have run out of luck
I feel that I have been betrayed
And I am up in arms, I am dismayed

I want my problems to be sorted out
I want everything resolved without a shadow of a doubt
I want my life to run smoothly
And I want to silence those who are accusatory

I need my faith in human nature to be renewed
I need to show that things have been misconstrued
I need the backing of my peers
And I need to demonstrate to them I am sincere

I can't carry on the way things are
I can't heal the wounds without leaving a scar
I can't move forward with my life
And I can't believe I am to be made a sacrifice

That leaves me with just one thing to say
Please intervene and don't delay
Because I can't take much more
My problems are real and can't be ignored

Apology

I think I am owed an apology
You have accused me quite wrongly
You have assumed that I have committed a crime
When it was someone else's error all the time
Why did you point your finger straight at me?
And take away what was left of my dignity
You have put me through hell
Just because I have been mentally unwell
You thought my illness made me deceitful
And consequently you never treated me as your equal
Now I demand respect from you
I want to be awarded the status I am due
Also, never underestimate my resilience
And bare in mind that I will out shine you with my
brilliance
I will always gain the upper hand
You will be subservient and I will be in command

At A Bad Time

You have caught me at a bad time
For I have lost those feelings so sublime
I have been thrown back into the mire
My numbers up, my health pass has expired
I am back on depression street
I am without a paddle stuck in that dried up creek
Who knows how long I will have to wait
Before the rain will allow me to once more navigate
Down the river of life
Following some sort of divine light
I trust I will only have to wait a short time
And I know good fortune will one day be mine
Until then I must be a patient patient
Still looking for the right reagents
To mix together in the correct proportions
In such a way as to stop this inner contortion
But I also know that by putting my feelings down on
paper
I have made a move towards ending this caper
Of course I will still need help from you out there
I will need your tender loving care
But I hope that eventually
I will be well for all perpetuity

Lying Here

Lying here on my bed
I quietly sob to myself
Thinking how cruel life is
And what an awful hand I have been dealt
Most of the time I soldier on
Keeping my chin up
But every once in a while
I find I come unstuck
Then I let it all out
I breakdown and cry
Releasing my pent up emotions
And giving a great big sigh
Afterwards I feel better though
The pressure in my head has relented
I am ready to do battle once more
Even if the agony seems endless
But I am an advocate of the saying
"If at first you don't succeed try, try again"
And I constantly remind myself
I must push on through the pain

Not Guilty

I am furious about how I have been treated
My anger is eating me up inside
You still believe I am guilty
Even when I have an alibi
You have dropped the charges
And have dismissed the allegations
But you continue to find it necessary
To slap down rules and regulations
You have threatened me
And said if I over step the mark
I will be in serious trouble
And I will be dealt with in a way that's harsh

Well I am not going to be bullied by you
I don't have to stand for this
Because I am the innocent party
And should never have been admonished
You want me to go quietly
But I am going to put up a fight
I will make sure justice has been done
I will prove to you that I am in the right

Work

I need to find a place that's safe
Away from this interminable rat race
I have pushed myself to the limit
But find that all I can do is plummet
Down from a great height
Because I can't keep up the fight
All the time I have let my job come first
I never put myself before work
Now something is going to have to give
A change is needed in the way I live
Otherwise I will crack up
And then everyone really would be stuck
The bottom line is the buck stops with me
If there is a problem then I will have to oversee
I will put the world to right
But hope I don't pay a terrible price
My health may suffer as a consequence
And there will be no form of recompense
I am the only person on whom I can rely
You certainly couldn't criticise me for being work shy!

Midlife Crisis

I have had my fortieth Birthday
It has been and gone
My face has extra lines
And grey hairs have come along
I look in the mirror
I don't like what I see
Who is this middle aged person
Staring back at me?
I am having a midlife crisis
I have lost my identity
I don't know where I am going
Or what is in store for me
I need to take stock
To reflect on what has passed
And analyse my achievements
Because the time has gone so fast
Many goals have been reached
Many dreams have been fulfilled
But would I have done things differently
If I had been more strong willed?
I can't live my life over
And change the things that went wrong
But now I have the opportunity
To get back on track where I belong
I can start with a clean sheet
And re-evaluate my targets
I can discard all my baggage
And flush it down the toilet
From now on I will be more focussed
I will be more determined to succeed
This midlife crisis may be beneficial after all
And a good kick up the backside is what I need

Post Natal Depression

I peer over the side of the cot
I see a baby that I have gently rocked
But she can't be my flesh and blood
Because I don't love her as I should
The bond between us has something missing
And I find this terribly distressing
I am at a loss as how to care for her
I have let her down, I am a complete failure
Will someone please take this baby away?
Or she will come to some harm I am afraid
I am feeling depressed, I have the baby blues
Nobody warned me that this situation could ensue
All I want is for someone to tell me
How to be a mother, a skill I thought came naturally

Illness

Although I have been sick for several months
Nobody has phoned me not even once
None of my friends have contacted me
I might as well have had leprosy
They have shied away because of my depression
Not realising I have a treatable condition
I would dearly love to chat with someone else
So I could explain to them just how I felt
Then they might start to understand
And possibly offer a helping hand
This would aid me to recover
And they would see I have an illness like any other

To My Doctor

Sometimes you don't want to believe me
When I say my life is a living hell
But deep in your heart you know
My behaviour only shows I am unwell
Don't judge me too harshly
I don't pretend to be what I am not
I have little control over my actions
Please don't put me on the spot
You never really knew me *before*
You don't know what I was like
But suffice it to say
Everyday was clear and bright
Now I have a continual battle
Against the forces of evil
Each day is a challenge
With much emotional upheaval
Despite taking the medication
I am not completely cured
My problems haven't gone away
Their view has just been slightly obscured
However I manage the best I can
For I still appreciate the simple things in life
Especially having children
And the love a husband gives his wife
So I apologise if you thought
I was asking too much of you
But sometimes I need your reassurance
And that's what pulls me through

HELP AND RECOVERY

Locked In

A momentary spark of understanding
A flicker of recognition
Still you are locked in your own thoughts
With no outward vision
I know making sense of it all
Is what you are trying to do
But there is no easy answer
Save waiting for a bolt out of the blue
It is very distressing to see you
Churning things over in your head
I long to reach you through the haze
And pull you into my world instead
Sometimes you are coherent
Which shows there is no brain damage
It is just a monumental feat for you to speak
It is more than you can manage
I pray you will soon return
For all I can do is watch patiently
But I know from experience you will recover
I believe that vehemently

Back

I want you back
I don't want to wait patiently
For every now and then
I see the 'real you' if only transiently
It is these little glimpses
That show you are still there inside
And this is what I hold onto
On this emotional rollercoaster ride
I am going to tough it out though
And give you my endless support
I know time helps in recovery
I only wish it could be bought
Let me hold you in my arms
And kiss you on the cheek
Let me tell you that you will get better
Things are improving as we speak

In Denial

Before you can be helped
You have to admit to being ill
It is a brave thing to do
But you must not be in denial
You have to recognise
That your behaviour has changed
You display little idiosyncrasies
Saying words that are rather strange
Once you have accepted
There is something wrong
Then you have made the first step toward recovery
Bearing in mind your journey may be long
Look at yourself closely
Are you ready to move forward?
Stop being in denial
It is a position that is so awkward

I Need You Now!

Sometimes you don't recognise
When I am in need
You seem to have your blinkers on
And I am not the first sight you see
You don't exactly ignore me
I am just not in the forefront of your mind
I know that you still care for me
And that you are trying to be kind
But every now and then
I require your full attention
Because I am hurting inside
I am in a turmoil of twisted emotion
If I could stop you in your tracks
If I could call for a time out
It would become obvious
What the problem is all about
I need you to protect me
From the thoughts inside my head
I need you to direct me
And put and end to the tears I shed
Please listen to me
For pity's sake
I need your help right now
It really cannot wait!

Sometimes

Sometimes you have to stop and reassess
Take a step back from your position if it is making you
depressed
You have to view things from a different angle
In order that your problems can be untangled
Then you can analyse what makes life worthwhile
And all the good things that make you want to smile
Like lazing in the summer sun
Under clear blue skies, it is second to none
Or watching your children as they laugh and play
Reminding you of your own carefree childhood days
A glass of wine shared with friends
Relaxing at the evenings end
So many reasons to make your time on earth
A place where working hard brings its just deserts
When I am ill it is to these thoughts I cling
Knowing that this will help me recover and ease my
suffering

How Can I Help?

How can I help you?
How can I set your wrongs to right?
I want you to feel better
But I don't know how to make the future bright
I am here beside you
Hoping you will tell me what to do
There must be a way to cure your ills
Something that will see you through
I feel that I am useless
Nothing I say gives you a lift
I don't understand why you have depression
And why it is so difficult to shift
I try to be patient
I get frustrated too you know
Everyone says it will take time
But it will eventually go
I hope their prognosis is correct
Because I want you back the way you used to be
I still love you with all my heart
But I need you loving me

Time to Mend

Don't let me down
Don't give me reason to frown
Now more than ever I need you around
To keep me safe and sound

Stay here with me
In my hour of need
Continue to give your love freely
For without you I am nobody

You are my greatest ally
You are the only one on whom I can rely
But still I don't want you to see me cry
Wait for me until I can dry my eyes

Stand by me to the bitter end
You are my last remaining friend
To you my shaking arms I extend
Hold me tight until I have time to mend

Help

Do you wake up early in the morning
Feeling sad and feeling blue?
Then I have got the remedy
I'll tell you what to do
Grab some paper and a pencil
Pull up a comfy chair
Listen to what I have to say
Because I have already been there
Make a list of all your troubles
Make a list of all your strife
We'll tackle them together
And we'll get you back your life
Where shall we begin?
Where shall we make a start?
What I think this boils down to
Is a problem of the heart
Your very soul is dying
You've lost just who you are
But let me help you back together
Let me heal those emotional scars
If we take it slowly
Just one step at a time
We can get things in order
And make everything rhyme
There is no quick fix
No miracle cure
But bit by bit we'll sort it out
And find the truth that's for sure
I hope this relieves the pressure
And eases the pain
Because there are other people in this world
Who are feeling just the same
So you don't have to suffer
Out there by yourself
I am here to be with you
I am here to help

The Forgotten Smile

Have you forgotten how to smile?
Does your life seem to be a continual trial?
Then I can empathise with you
Because I have to admit I've been there too
In depression is the most awful place to be
And as one who knows I offer my sympathy
But it doesn't have to be like this forever
There is a way to make things better
To start with you have to ask for help
Stop bottling it up and chastising yourself
You need to express your fears
And maybe even shed a few tears
Then the healing process can begin
You can change the predicament you're in
The first step is the hardest one to take
But I know how so I'll demonstrate
You just put one foot in front of the other
To work through your problems in an orderly manner
Instead of seeing them with negative connotations
You begin to add more positive associations
For each task you do manage to achieve
Congratulate yourself that you did succeed
This will boost your confidence
And you will benefit from the difference
At times you will still feel very low
But these will diminish and eventually go
Your life will get back on the rails
It is tried and trusted method that for me never fails
Then one day you will catch yourself smiling
It is an expression that is so beguiling

Rescue

You seem mentally stranded
Trapped in a world of your own
But I am here to rescue you
With this rope I've thrown
Tie the rope tightly
In a knot around your waist
And I will pull you up
To a place that's safe
I am able to do this
Because I understand your plight
I have been in that same dark pit
But eventually found the light
I don't want you to suffer
When there are many things I can do to help
I know implicitly how you are feeling
You don't have to explain yourself
With a little guidance from me
We can start to turn things around
You must listen to what I have to say
If the route to recovery is to be found
I recommend you take the drugs on offer
Because they are very beneficial
The doctor isn't trying to poison you
You are not a lamb that's sacrificial
Then I will teach you
The Art of Distraction
Where you force yourself to do things
Even though they have no attraction
Momentarily your mood will be lifted
The bad thoughts will subside or disappear
And while you're are focussed on the job in hand
Your subconscious brain will gradually clear
In this way you will slowly put back
All the jigsaw puzzle pieces
And you will become whole again
Your world will once more be completed

Unfortunately there are no short cuts
It will take a while to work things through
You will have to remain resolute
But then time itself is a great healer too

Dry Your Eyes

Dry your eyes because
I am here to rid you of your pain
I understand the hurt you are feeling
But I know you are not going insane
Focus on what I am saying
You have to make an effort to help yourself
I can only point you in the right direction
The rest has to come from you and no one else
The drugs that you will be given
Are to relieve the symptoms you display
Like the early morning waking
And the constant anxiety
They will not cure the root cause of your depression
But your thinking will start to clear
Then you will be able to address your problems
And tackle your illness no matter how severe
Also talk to those who care for you
Discuss the best course of action
You will quickly find
That you get a positive reaction
I am glad you have stopped crying
Let me wipe away your last tear
Better times are approaching
They are so very near

Saved

Be strong and never give in
One day you will surely win
I know that you are suffering
But I urge you to keep trying

For just on the horizon
A new day has begun
And all your strength must be summoned
In order that your problems can be overcome

Today is the day to start your recovery
To tread the path to self discovery
A time to set aside all your worries
But don't panic there is no need to hurry

I will lead you every step of the way
I will guide you so that you don't go astray
Together we will climb the barricades
And you can shout out "My Life Has Been Saved"

The Carer

I am a carer for
Someone who is mentally ill
I have had no proper training
I don't know if I fit the bill
But I have no choice because
It is my loved one who is in need
They have become a shadow of their former selves
And have become very withdrawn indeed
All I can do is
Carry on as normal
Imposing structure on the day
Without it becoming too formal
I have to cajole them
Into participating in the daily tasks
Instead of just sitting there
With every moment more daunting than the last
I talk to them continuously
To stop them retreating into their inner space
Sometimes it is necessary
To deny them time to contemplate
Encouragement and direction
Are what are required from me
I have to take control
Although I mustn't become too pushy
I have to be patient
Yet determined not to let depression defeat me too
I must remain a rock
And I will have to see things through
In this way I pray that I can
Ease the suffering and the pain
I want my loved one to recover
I don't want my efforts to have been in vain

Two Steps Forward

To recover from mental illness is often
Two steps forward and one step back
Your progress won't be linear
And there are likely to be set backs
But when you analyse things overall
You'll see improvement is being made
And you can chalk off all the miles stones
As you pass them along the way
A safety net will be put in place
By those who really care
Professionals, friends and relatives
Who want to rid you of your despair
The pattern of your life will gradually change
Your problems won't seem so huge
And now that there is this safety net
You may find it will never need to be used

Neural Networks

The working of the mind
Is very intricate
With its neural networks
That are so elaborate
Theory has it
That in the normal brain
Neural networks are constantly being built up
And then broken down again
But what happens when
You are suffering from depression?
Well, a large network become fixated
Against your own discretion
You have no control

But these networks must be broken down
Medication and counselling can help
And will clear your face of that frown
Once you have broken the negative cycle
You can start on the road to rehabilitation
Hopefully you will swiftly recover
And begin to see things with appreciation

Today

Today was a wasted day
Nothing was done that was constructive
I couldn't find an occupation
Or anything that was productive
In consequence I feel a little useless
For I have nothing to show for my time
But wait a minute!
Surely I have committed no crime
Haven't I made it through the day?
That must be an achievement in itself
Considering my mental state of play
And that I am trying to manage all by myself
A few weeks ago
I couldn't have coped on my own
I would be constantly seeking support
Even if it was merely talking on the phone
Things are improving then
Progress is being made
I just have to take it slowly
Day by single day

Therapy

I think cognitive therapy can be useful
But it is not the answer lets be truthful
I very strongly believe
That the correct neurotransmitter is the key
Once you have the right chemicals in your brain
Then your mind can start to take the strain
Of course you still need support
To put in order all your thoughts
But in the end it is down to you
To find the strength that will pull you through
Drug therapy has been my salvation
I am living proof and a vindication

Rallying Cry

There is no use crying over spilt milk
Or the flowers in the vase as they begin to wilt
These are things we cannot change
We cannot rewind and start again
Therefore don't look back, don't dwell on the past
Keep pushing forward for life is moving fast
Focus your mind on what is ahead
But don't project the future as something to dread
You must give a rallying cry
And stand your ground for you must not be denied
If you are worried that you can't make it on your own
Remember help is at hand you don't need to be alone
You must cast aside depression, you must break the
mould
It is finally time to come in from the cold

Eliminated

There is no future
There is no past
I am stuck in limbo
With its torture unsurpassed

There is no way out
There is no emergency exit
I am trapped with my own thoughts
My attempts to escape are ineffective

There is only doom
There is only depression
Unless I can find help
To make things change direction

There must be a route to follow
There must a path with saving graces
And I will beg, steal and borrow
If this will leave my depression eliminated

What Can I Say?

What can I say
To make the blues go away?
Nothing will ease the intense pain
That is generated within your brain
Outwardly you look no different
But your suffering is inherent
Of a serious mind malfunction
And this has left you with a feeling of compunction
I can throw words of comfort your direction
But none will lead to an instant correction
Of the chemicals inside your head
That would leave your depression defeated
What I can say is this
'You' are sorely missed
Hold on for in time your brain will heal
And you will no longer feel
That your life has come to an end
Eventually you will be on the mend
Just as with any other disease
Your body will fight to overcome the discrepancies

Learning to cope

When life is going badly
When life isn't going too great
You need to get some coping strategies
That you can put in place
You should contact a professional
Or even just a friend
So you can discuss the best plan
One on which you can depend
They will record that you are feeling down
And don't know which way to turn
But they will also want to know your troubles
And if there is any more to learn
Together you will formulate
The best things to do
This should ease the burden
And give better direction to you
It may not work immediately
And at times it will still be hard to cope
But you have to hang on in there
Because there is always hope!

Magic Potion

If there was one thing I could give to you
Do you know what it would be?
It would be a magic potion
That would put an end to your misery
It would remove that empty feeling
And the thought that life is pointless
You would no longer dread the future
Or feel that you were completely useless
It would boost your self esteem
It would restore your self belief
The feeling of trepidation would evaporate
You would stop shaking like a leaf

117

The dark cloud hanging over you
Would be blown away
It would be a remedy for life
And would ensure that good times were here to stay
I would call my witches brew
'The Essence of Liberation'
And it would transform your world
Into a place of great expectation
Should such a magic potion be perfected
You will be the first to know
Because it will be a very powerful weapon
Banishing depression from all your tomorrows

Art of Distraction

Tell me why
You have to cry?
Is it the mixed up thoughts
That spiral round more than they ought?
Somehow you have to break through
And start to put these feelings behind you
You have to use the art of distraction
Where you force yourself to do things that have no
attraction
But these terrible thoughts will briefly disappear
While the task involves you and your thinking clears
When it is over you can praise yourself for succeeding
Even if progress is slow you are still achieving
Bit by bit, day by day
You will eventually find the way
For all the pain will have gone
And your heart will once more be filled with song

Rapport

I met someone today
With whom I had an immediate rapport
We both suffer from depression
And I instantly knew we shared a common lore
I would never wish mental illness on anyone
But it is comforting to know
That there are other people
Who know how the story goes
If you have never been struck down yourself
You can only try to imagine what it is like
It is very difficult to explain
Or find words that will suffice
We sufferers stick together
Because we have a deep understanding
We give each other support
Especially when life can be so very demanding
A friendly face, a hand to hold
Reassurance and a caring smile
These are all things we can give to others
And that we may need ourselves just once in a while

The Future

What is to become of me?
Do I have a future?
I don't know what fate will bring
But I pray there won't be too much torture
My sentence has been served
I have paid my dues
This depressive phase is over
And I am no longer subdued
I am picking up the pieces
Of my tattered past
Trying to rebuild my world
And take things firmly in my grasp
Slowly I am moving forward
I am taking control
But it is still early days
And I am only out on parole
I hope that one day soon
I will be back with my friends and family
A job would be a bonus
But I will have to wait and see
Looking ahead and making plans
Doesn't seem so daunting
And maybe there will come a time
When it will be my good fortune that I'm flaunting
Whatever is in store for me
I will never forget this episode
But now I am ready to continue
Down life's long and winding road

Optimism

I am an eternal optimist
I can always see the world in a favourable light
Even when the chips are down
I believe that things will turn out alright
You will never dampen my spirits
Or put the mockers on what I am doing
Life is there to be enjoyed
In whatever activity you are pursuing
I know that a certain amount of luck
Is required to help you on your way
But sometimes you can make your own
Just by being positive in what you say
Take a leaf out of my book
Don't hesitate to make that leap of faith
Go where your heart is drawing you
And you will find everything else will fall into place

Special Friend

They say pride comes before a fall
And it must be true because I have hit a brick wall
My life was racing along full of purpose
When suddenly I became incredibly nervous
A part of my mental capability had gone
The part that copes with whatever comes along
I had lost the capacity to plan and look ahead
Even the simplest tasks were faced with fear and
dread
Once I even found myself collapsed at the foot of the
stairs
Feeling all alone and overcome with despair
You can imagine then the relief I felt
When someone knocked at the door offering help
They told me that my life was not about to end
And that they had come to be a special kind of friend
The sort who would listen and understand
And then would take me by the hand
To lead me to a place that was safe
Somewhere we could contemplate my fate
They were true to their word
And gave me a chance to be heard
This allowed me to have better insight
And showed me how to start to put my world to right
Now I know I have this guardian angel
It gives me the strength to turn the tables
For I have faith that they will rescue me
If I were ever in desperate need
But do you know this friend so true?
Why of course, because this friend is you

Stop and Think

My pen has just run out of ink
So now is a good time to stop and think
Is your life proceeding as you would wish?
Tell the truth be completely honest
If the answer is 'Yes' then you can breathe a sigh of
relief
But if not then you can talk to me I'll be discreet
Tell me what is troubling you
Have you lost track of what you are supposed to do?
I recommend you don't dwell too much on the past
Learn to live for today because it goes so fast
Also don't worry about what the future holds
Let things develop and find their own way to unfold
But still look out for opportunities and try to remain
astute
You can always reach your goals even if it is not by the
tried and tested route
Now buck up your ideas and get up from that easy
chair
Grab what life has on offer make the most of the world
out there

Here and Now

I was severely depressed
And my feelings were hard to express
I suffered and was terribly distressed
So much so I thought I would have cardiac arrest

But now I feel there is hope
I am sure I will find a way to cope
And I will stop myself slipping down that slope
I will be able to remove the noose from around my
throat

Deep inside I know I don't really want to die
A part of me still wants to be alive
I will therefore continue to strive
Knowing that soon the pain will start to subside

Eventually the sun will break through the clouds
And for you watching in the crowd
I will stand up tall and proud
I will be back in the here and now

A Happier Place

When you are depressed
Everything becomes a monumental task
You would rather sit in a chair
And not join in, even when asked
The world is whizzing around you
At break neck speed
And you feel unable to take part
Because you have lost the will to succeed
But things can change
You just need a little help with motivation
One tiny step is all it takes
To set the ball rolling in the right direction
Then slowly but surely
You will gather some positive momentum
The goal posts will be shifted in your favour
And you can re-align the equilibrium
If you take this approach
You will find that you can keep pace
And your world will have turned into
A brighter happier place

Discovery

I have made a startling discovery
That hopefully will help me on the road to recovery
I have found that if I externalise my thoughts
Then living doesn't appear to be so fraught
When I record my brainwaves in the form of text
This stops me from becoming overly vexed
It allows me to rationalise my feelings
And makes what life has to offer that much more
appealing
It also enables me to take a step back
To see my problems in a way that is more detached
And things that seem insurmountable at first glance
Become more easily rectified given half a chance
Writing down my thoughts brings order out of chaos
For me it is the answer but then I am completely
biased

Salty Tears

These salty tears I cry
Are not shed in anguish
I no longer have to sit here
In my jail and languish

These salty tears I cry
Are of joy rather than pain
For my life is back on the rails
And I can join in once again

These salty tears I cry
Started so long ago
It seems like an eternity
And looking back brings so much sorrow

These salty tears I cry
I brush away with my hand
But I don't wipe away the smile
I have made it to the promised land

Rain Rain Go Away

Rain
Rain
Go away
And don't come back on another day
This is the chant I am singing
Heralding a new beginning
For oak trees out of little acorns grow
And I am sowing some seeds of hope for tomorrow
It is never too late to initiate change
But I will be careful to keep the targets within range
I will be cautious and pace myself
So that I don't have to rely on others too much for help
I will become more self sufficient
And therefore even more resilient
To the knocks that occur in life
I will be able to cope
If lightening strikes

Bravery

That first step to start my recovery
Required a certain amount of bravery
I was frightened I would not make it
And was sure I would make a big mistake of it
But that didn't happen I did succeed
I found the courage and a little self belief
What did I do next?
Of course, I took a second step
This seemed a bit easier than the first
And restored some of my self worth
The third step still required some bravery
But I knew nothing would turn out to be unsavoury
The fourth step convinced me I would survive
And I no longer needed to run away and hide
Then the fifth, sixth and seventh
Boosted my self confidence
The next few days began to gather pace
I realised I had managed to escape
Now I don't have to count off the days
And I can shout out "Hip Hip Hooray!"

Feeling Well

Today is the start of a new chapter in my life
I have decided to banish all my strife
From now on I am going to be happy
The glass is going to be half full instead of half empty
I am going to make positive moves
And turn things around so they improve
The pieces of my world are coming together
I feel I have ridden out the stormy weather
My inner strength has won through
And I know exactly what to do
I have purpose, I have drive
I am finally starting to feel alive

The misery I felt before
Has vanished and is no more
The mental anguish which used to dominate every
waking moment
Has been replaced by shear contentment
I can't explain how things have altered
But I pray I never falter
I want to be well all the time
Because these feelings are so sublime

Survivor

I am a survivor
Just hanging on by my finger tips
Mentally battered by my ordeal
Bruised by my mind's own tricks
I have come out the other side
From the darkness into the light
The sun is warm upon my face
Adding further strength to win the fight
In the end it is my own willpower
That has caused the barometer to change
Helped by those who care for me
And who influenced my thoughts to rearrange
I don't know how much time has elapsed
To reach this position
But this feeling of well being
Is a very enjoyable acquisition
I tread cautiously though
Not trying to run before I can walk
But knowing that the effort I put in
Will reap it's own rewards

My World

I wake up each morning safe in my bed
Looking forward with anticipation to the day ahead
Planning what I am going to do
Instead of feeling that I haven't got a clue
Maybe work today will give me inspiration
Or at the very least some sort of job satisfaction
If not, then I am sure I'll find
Happiness in caring for others and being kind
Of course my most important roles in life
Are being a loving mother and a loyal wife
The hours my family spend together
Really do give me such enormous pleasure
I can always picture my children in the sun
Playing games and having fun
I love my husband with all my heart
And pray we never have to be apart
I have also learned to love myself
Although at times I have needed help
Here is my world, it is a colourful space
Full of hope and joy, such a wondrous place

Life Conception

The trade winds are set fair
I am enjoying life I do declare
Once more I am on an even keel
The world has become so surreal
Suddenly I find
My depression has been left far behind
The old pattern has been broken
A new language will now be spoken
One that reiterates the positives
And does away with all the negatives

I will make sure I don't relapse
I won't allow myself to again collapse
Because by altering the way I perceive
The ups and downs, I believe
I won't lay myself open to depression
I have changed my life conception

Change

Something incredible has happened
And it has happened to me
A pathway in my brain has clicked
I have been shocked back into reality
Instead of wallowing in self pity
I can see the error of my ways
My problems can be resolved
And my sanity can be saved
I am ready to help my self
To correct the abnormalities
New hope has been ignited
And the future holds endless possibilities
What has changed is quite dramatic
It was as if there was a missing link
I don't know how my brain has altered
But I know it has brought me back from the brink
I feel totally different
I have been given a new lease of life
I am going to take this opportunity
To set my world to right

The Tide Has Turned

The tide has turned
All my ships have come in
I am thankful to be alive
To enjoy what is happening
I have been unburdened
A great weight has been lifted
The future is looking bright
My depression has finally shifted
It didn't happen overnight
The change developed gradually
Good days started to out number bad
And now I find I can live quite happily
I can't see why I had such trouble
Being alive and just surviving
But now I am no longer depressed
I have surfaced from those depths that I was diving
I am a different person
There has been an alteration to my inner core
Little hills are enough for me to conquer
I don't need to move mountains anymore
I have scaled down my ambitions
And now set myself less challenging goals
I take pleasure in the simple things
That is all I need to make me whole

Goals

I have many goals in life
But this can make things awkward
I am always busy
And being constantly driven forward
Whether I am playing sport
Or just doing the washing up
My mind is often racing
Dreaming of that trophy cup
I am continuously striving
To be the very best
I want to get my nose in front
And beat all the rest
Ultimately I want to win
I need to come in first
Because this power that is within me
Is almost fit to burst
If I channel all this strength
That is locked up inside of me
Then the sky's the limit
And who knows what I can achieve
One day I will get there
And my quest will be complete
But what will I do then
With this energy that's replete?
I will have to store it up
And try to be content
Until I let some more out
Through the overflow vent

A cautionary note:
I will have to be a little careful though
To only do what I am able
Otherwise I'll set unrealistic goals
At a level that's unattainable

A WORLD OF LOVE

Our Home

Originally our house was little bigger than a caravan
With no space to swing a cat or hide away the pans
But with the passing years things have really changed
And we have expanded again and again
The kitchen is small but very neat
It has everything I need to make the meals complete
Our family tries to eat together once a day
To discuss our problems and have our say
We do all this in our family space
That is a large and very airy place
We have a beautiful garden that gives us endless
pleasure
Some where we can relax and enjoy at our leisure
Each bedroom is used in a different way
According to the time of day
My son's room is for homework and entertaining
friends
Then finally sleep at the evening's end
Whereas my daughter's room has seen the greatest
transition
And now incorporates a sofa, piano and a television
My bedroom is where I go to as a sanctuary
But it is also a place for loving and for intimacy
We have two bathrooms now that's a plus
It means we can all get ready when we're in a rush
My home is very important, important to me
And I will show it off for everyone to see

Our World

Our world is a land of opportunity
It is a place we can live with relative impunity
The way it revolves should be seen with incredulity
And we should take care of it that is our responsibility

Our world is constantly being adapted to suit our needs
We can alter it and change the way it is perceived
It is somewhere that our dreams can be achieved
While providing enough space for everyone to breathe

Our world is a place that we should hold sacred
It always provides us with our daily bread
We wouldn't want to leave or live anywhere else
instead
And if God actually made it he should be congratulate

Smile

Looking at a clear blue sky
On a summer's day
Watching children run about
When they are at play
Eating a meal with friends
As they gather round
Finding something you have lost
When you thought it would never be found
Giving your love and care
To your family
Brightening someone else's life
And causing them to be happy
There really are so many reasons
To make you want to smile
These are the moments you should cherish
Because they make everything worthwhile

The World

Sometimes I get up early
To watch the sunrise in the east
It is a time of tranquillity
The world is still at peace
As I look out from the veranda
And lean against the rail
I can see great shafts of light
Shooting from a sun that is oh so pale
The horizon is quite misty
And there is a morning dew
I try to capture the moment
Everything has a rosy hue
This is the part of the day
When no one else is around
I am completely alone
Only my breathing makes a sound
I dwell on the miracle of my existence
And the enormity of it all
How was the world created?
It only took seven days if I recall

Hope

There will always be hope
A way to move forward, a way to cope
Recovery is within everyone's scope
Even though at times life is no joke

There will always be help at hand
People who will care for their fellow man
Others who will understand
How hard life is with all it's demands

There will always be someone to catch us if we fall
People who will make us feel special
Others who will sort out our inner turmoil
And stop our lives from being spoiled

The Cycle of Love

Love is all around us
In everything we do
It starts before we are born
It begins when we are in the womb
Our parents nurture us as babies
Their love has no bounds
They will care for us forever
No matter what blemishes are found
Naturally we give our love back
We shouldn't take our parents for granted
They provide a solid base
In which our feet are firmly planted
Then we can go out into the world
To find other people to love
Those we find attractive
And who fit us like a glove
How we choose who to fall in love with
Is difficult to predict
Certain traits are more appealing
And they need to match our wish list
But there is someone out there for all of us
Of that you can be assured
And hopefully there will be one special love
The type that will endure
Then we can create a new life
To begin the pattern again
We become the parents
And the cycle of love is sustained

Love

I love my family
I love my friends
They make my life secure
I can depend on them
I love my work
I love my sport
They make my world
A place with rich rewards
I love myself
I love who I am
Everything is wonderful
It is all going to plan
But I stop just for a second
To ask the question why
I should be so lucky
When others can only cry?
All I can do is live
My life to the full
And try to ease the suffering
Of those whose lives are cruel
If I can brighten
Someone else's day
By a few kind words
Said in the right way
Then I will be satisfied
I will be happy with myself
Knowing that I have made a difference
And that I have truly help

My Family

Let me check if the coast is clear
It is so I can tell you something I hold most dear
My family is the most important thing in my life
For them I would make the ultimate sacrifice
They come first and above all else
I will always be on hand to offer them help
I will love them unconditionally
And I will defend them in the face of adversity
No one will be allowed to split us up
We are joined by a bond that is really tough
If all our material things were taken away
We would still be together come what may
I can't imagine life without my family
The world would become cold and meaningless to me

My love for my Children

You bring me such happiness
You often reward me with your kiss
The love you give is boundless
And I know that I am truly blessed

I love to watch the games you play
Especially outside upon a summer's day
But even when the weather has put paid
I never wish to send you away

You make my life complete
You lift me to the highest level I can reach
And with every heart beat
I realise your very existence is a miraculous feat

My Children

I have two children
A girl and a boy
I treasure them most dearly
They are my pride and joy
Every day I thank God
For sending them to me
I will take good care of them
And love them tenderly
In my eyes
They can do no wrong
And I will defend them
With my love so strong
I will comfort them
In their time of need
I will standby them
And encourage them to succeed
My love for them is never in question
It will never be in doubt
It is what being a parent
Is really all about

Children

Pregnancy is a special
And exciting time for you
With the weight of expectation
As one being becomes two
The actual birth may be difficult
And really hard to bare
But in the end you get what you've been waiting for
A baby delivered to your care
In the beginning they are demanding
With many a sleepless night
A time when you can only give your love
And hope you get it right
In the first year they change so quickly
They change so very fast
They are becoming tiny people
And you must make the moment last
Next comes a harder time
When they really test you out
Often driving you up the wall
Making you want to scream and shout
All too soon they're off to school
They can manage more on their own
You have to cut those apron strings
Or they'll never be full grown
They are getting older now,
They've turned into your little friend
But they continue to need your love and help
You're still their parents in the end
Finally they leave the nest
To make their lives of course
But you are in the background
To give them guidance and support
Children are very rewarding
They give you unconditional love
I think they are made in heaven
And are sent by God above

Thank You for my Children

My children are my source of inspiration
Although at times they cause me much consternation
Making me want to shout at them
While questioning where I would be without them
Just yesterday I was cradling them in my arms
Protecting them from any harm
Back then they seemed so delicate
I wrapped them up so they wouldn't break
As the years have passed I have had to let go
I have had to give them room to grow
While trying to cement a friendship that would really
last
And wishing that the time wouldn't go so fast
I have pushed, directed, guided them
To be the best they possibly can
I adore them now as much as ever
They are still my little treasures
And if there is a God on high
I thank him for all the love I have derived

Marriage

The sanctity of marriage
Has stood the test of time
Even in our jet set world
It is still part of our grand design
We all want to find a partner
Someone with whom to share our lives
We need their physical contact
Which strengthens the emotional ties
To make this commitment
We must be absolutely certain
It can be a scary process
But you will know when you have found the right
person
The future becomes clear
And it is filled with love
Two people become conjoined
Made for each other by God above
When the marriage vows are spoken
There can be no going back
You have to give your all
And protect your relationship from attack
Marriage is forever
It goes on for time in memoriam
Although it is a serious business
Never fear, it is the greatest fun

My Husband

I fell in love with my husband
It was love at first sight
I knew from the very start
That I had chosen right
I wanted to spend every moment together
And share his company
He had this sort of magic
That made me feel all tingley
Our bond grew ever stronger
With the passage of time
And finally we got married
Confirming this love of mine
We are the best of friends now
As well as being lovers
And yet with each new day
There is still more to discover
This friendship is very special
This link is very tight
I really need my husband
I love him with all my might

You

I love you
And you love me
Together with our two kids
We make the nuclear family
I thank my lucky stars
That I met you when I did
Back then we were merely children
Living at home completely cosseted
But we struck out together
Into the big wide world
To make our indelible mark
And to watch our lives unfurl
We have built a home
Which we have furnished with love
Despite our lack of money
We have each other and that's enough
I understand your thinking
We share common goals
And also share our problems
To you I can bare my soul
The children have brought us even closer
They are our flesh and blood
We nurture them effectively
And see them develop as they should
My life with you is perfect
I don't want anything to change
I am still captivated by you
Now isn't that so strange?

Look

Look how far we have come
Look how we have developed since we were young
I am sure I made the right decision
I had a sort of premonition

Look at all we have achieved
Look at our home and our family
I am sure we couldn't have done any better
We have made things perfect and to the letter

Look how closely we have become entwined
Look how your hand fits neatly into mine
I am sure we were destined to always be together
I know I will love you forever and ever

My Love For You

I often think of you when we're apart
For there is a yearning in my heart
We have become so closely knit
More important than any other friendship
You support me when times are tough
You are my diamond in the rough
When I am down you put back my smile
With your boyish playful style
Together we make a strong team
Enabling us to live out our dreams
I can stand proudly by your side
Knowing that our thoughts will coincide
My love for you will never end
That is the one thing on which you can depend

Sorry

I am sorry
So sorry for being me
I know I have let you down
That is plain to see
I am sorry I haven't lived
Up to your expectations
I may have promised much
But that was purely speculation
You fell in love
With someone you thought was strong
A person who was confident
And never got things wrong
Well this has all changed
Because of my mental illness
I have had to lean on you
In my many times of crisis
I have really put
Our marriage vows to the test
And yet you have stood by me
Both in health and in sickness
I am very fortunate
That you didn't pack your bags and leave
You have never doubted who I am
You have always given me a reprieve
I thank you then
For being my husband and my best friend
One day I promise to pay you back
With an added dividend

Bite Your Tongue

You never criticise me
You never raise your voice
Even when you think I'm wrong
You bite your tongue out of choice
We seldom argue
Because you just turn away
I can bait you all I like
But you don't rise up to what I say
You are always patient with me
When I rant and rave
You don't tell me to shut up
Or learn to behave
I know I can be difficult
But luckily you are very tolerant too
You soak up all the punches
That I level at you
Please don't change your stance
For without you where would I be?
There would be no one left
To look after me

My Love

I love to touch your face
Draw my fingers across your lips
It is very sensual
This stimulation at the tips
I love to run my hands through your hair
And up and down your back
You are all strong and smooth
I can feel where your muscles are attached
I love your arms to hold me
In a close embrace
I love to kiss your neck
And enjoy your special taste

You are the only one I need
To keep me safe and warm
I love to snuggle up to you
And wake together at the break of dawn
You are my soul mate
Someone I can trust implicitly
I can share everything with you
Knowing that you love me

My Heart

My heart is pounding in my chest
As you casually approach
The palms of my hands are damp with sweat
And I can feel a lump in my throat
Your mere presence sends my pulse racing
The smell of you excites
I tell myself to stay calm and collected
But I can't control my sexual appetite
You are my dream come true
The answer to all my prayers
If I had more time
I would simply stop and stare
Then you brush up close
And kiss me on the cheek
You take my breathe away
I am unable to speak
Every moment spent with you
Is pure unadulterated pleasure
I will never take you for granted
You are my most valuable treasure

Boys Night Out

Here I am in my bed all alone
Waiting for my husband to come home
He has gone out drinking with his mates
And as usual he won't be in the house till rather late
I worry a little that he will come to some harm
And I dread that call to say there is cause for alarm
I know he needs time to be with his friends
But I also know he will return to me in the end
I am a central part in his life
And that is why we are husband and wife
I won't be able to sleep till he is back
There is no way I can completely relax
I will just have to lie here on my side of the bed
And try to stop fretting that he is elsewhere instead

Infidelity

My marriage has lost its purity
My marriage has lost its security
My marriage has lost what it ought to be
Because I have broken my vow of fidelity

Why did I sleep with someone I barely know?
Why did I fall into this relationship that is so shallow?
Why was I unfaithful? I don't know
But now I have started it is hard to let it go

I have been found out, I have run out of luck
I have pressed the button for self destruct
I have become appalled at my own conduct
And now I find I have come unstuck

I must stop before I fall
I must put an end to it all
I must set things back as I recall
Before you label me a criminal

I hope that you can be forgiving
I hope you can see that without you my life's not worth
living
I hope that our marriage is worth saving
Because I am truly sorry I have been misbehaving

A Plea

My sweet love who was made in heaven
Hallowed be your name
For the veil of lies and deceit I've woven
Make me hang my head in shame
You are the only one who can
Forgive me of these sins
I plead with you to let me start over
Let me show there is still good within
If I am allowed to follow
What is right and true
I can regain your respect
And prove I can be faithful to you
Give me a second chance
Which I promise I won't disgrace
I will demonstrate my sincerity
And assure you that your love hasn't been misplaced

Forgive Me

I am sorry for what I have done
I am full of remorse
My behaviour has been deplorable
But now I want to chart a different course
I hope that you can forgive me
And that I can start a new
I want so desperately to be loved
By a love that comes from you

How Much?

How much do I love you?
Well let's just stop and see
I love you with all my heart
From here to infinity
With each passing day
My love for you increases
Without you my world would lose all meaning
It would simply fall to pieces
I rely on you
To stop me becoming too emotional
You keep my feet firmly on the ground
Pointing out what's rational
I am completely enwrapped
By your tender loving care
If you were to go away
It would be more than I could bear
Please stay by my side forever
For you have become the better half of me
We will live together in paradise
And be the envy of everyone we see

Your Love

I need a friend
Someone who is steadfast and true
I need a friend
Someone just like you

I need to be loved
By someone who is pure of heart
I need to be loved
And I want it to be you who plays that part

I need to be supported
By someone who will be my rock
I need to be supported
And I want you to release my shackles locked

You hold the key
That will make my future secure
You hold the key
That will enable my life to be enjoyed rather than
endured

Shear Contentment

You are a breath of fresh air to me
Like a summer's day with a gentle breeze
Your very presence lifts me like a kite
Soaring way up high and out of sight
I take such enormous pleasure
In being, just you and I, together
I want this time to be fixed in my memory
So that in the future I can remember how we used to
be
Young of heart and pure of mind
Living our lives without any confines
And I will savour this precious moment
That brings with it this feeling of shear contentment

In Love With You

Lay your head upon my pillow
Wrap yourself around me like the willow
Whisper sweet nothings in my ear
Tell me all the words of love I long to hear
You mesmerise me, you have me in raptures
And I am ready to be captured
By your web of adoration
That defies all measure or computation
All day I have been rehearsing this scenario
Over and over in my head it goes
And now the moment has arrived
When we can join our bodies and come alive
Afterwards I feel rejuvenated
For your love has left me elated
I pinch myself to see if it is all true
Yes I am in love, in love with you

My Daughter

My daughter was born
Ten years ago
And with each passing year
She has continued to grow
She has matured into
My little mate, my little friend
Now she is a person in her own right
Someone on whom I can depend
She has my respect
And she respects me too
Arguments are rare
There is seldom a hullabaloo
I treat her as a young adult
But still give her cuddles and a kiss
And although she is very independent
The time spent together I wouldn't miss
My daughter is very beautiful
She is a blue eyed blond
And I am very fortunate
To have this special mother daughter bond

Mother

You gave me life
And brought me into this world safely
You showed me love
The sort that is given spontaneously

You continued throughout my childhood
To give me your protection
You always understood me
And pointed me in the right direction

You wiped away the tears
When I tripped and fell
You cheered me up
When things weren't going too well

You have been there
In my times of greatest need
You have pushed me onwards
Willing me to succeed

You and I are now the best of friends
Together we share the fondest memories
And I want you to know
That as my mother you are exemplary

My Parents

My parents have always spoiled me
They have indulged my every whim
They have never made me go without
And I hope this is not a mortal sin
As a child they gave me pocket money
And provided toys and games
I think I was appreciative
And gave them my love in exchange
Of course they didn't just give me material things
They also gave me their love and affection
But stopped me doing anything stupid
Which I know was for my own protection
My parents have always supported me
In whatever venture I have undertaken
But they also forced me to do things I didn't like
If I am not very much mistaken
Now that I am grown up
I have a family of my own
I have learned my parenting skills from them
And I don't have to be shown
On reflection my parents have been excellent
The very best money can buy
I couldn't have asked for more from them
All my needs have been supplied

My Son

My son is very fashion conscious
He is particular about his clothes
They must have designer labels
Despite having to pay through the nose
It is not only the trousers and shirts
That must be just right
The boxer shorts require careful selection
And must be of a special type
He is also choosy about
What he puts on his feet
Especially when it comes to trainers
Even though he is no athlete
Then there is the personal hygiene
That must be catered for
He likes expensive perfume
To add a certain allure
His hair must be perfect
And cut in a trendy style
He has to have it highlighted
To look like he has been in the sun for a while
This behaviour is very expensive
He has been told money doesn't grow on trees
And that he had better get a well paid job
If he is to afford all these luxuries

Operation

My son is having an operation
To remove a tumour from his face
All the cancer will be removed
Leaving no cells left to annihilate
It will not be able then
To re-grow or re-invade
He will be left with a nice neat scar
That in time will fade
It is his choice to have the surgery
We have discussed all the options
And this appears to be
The best course of action
We have all faith in the surgeon
His expertise is second to none
He will keep us well informed
And hopefully nothing will go wrong
But it should be plain sailing
The doctors reassure us of that
And afterwards my boy won't need to hide his face
Underneath his baseball hat

Unrequited Love

It is raining in my heart
Because it is time for me to depart
But you have no idea that I love you
I keep my feelings hidden and out of view
If you were to know you may be shocked
And the foundations of our friendship would be rocked
But I want there to be more
Can't you feel the emotional draw?
I long for you to take me in your arms
And comfort me with all your worldly charms
I am not looking for sexual gratitude
All I yearn for is a change in attitude
Where you acknowledge me into your inner sanctum
To allow me to move with complete freedom
In you I find my intellectual equal
A sparring partner with whom to duel
You have also been there in my times of crisis
When I have been prone to cry at the very slightest
But I have to keep you at arms length
Which, requires all my self control and strength
And even though when we meet I still get excited
I know my love must remain unrequited

Disappointment and Decency

Many people find that in their lives
The world is full of disappointment no matter how hard
they try
And their reason to persevere has now been lost
For here they are down and out on their luck
But how can they rise above it all?
To stand aloof, to stand up tall?
In my opinion it has to start from love
A love that God has given to each and everyone of us
I don't mean you have to go to church each week
Or sing in the choir, or even preach
It is more about learning the rules of conduct
A building of a moral order that can't destruct
Care for the young, care for the old
Living in a community with shared goals
And if you give freely a little love to those in need
Kindness will be bestowed on you for having shown
common decency

Our Garden

A tranquil place
Where we can put our feet up
Bask in the sun
Sipping coffee from a cup
Or we can be active
Nurturing the flowers in the beds
Maybe grow some vegetables
To put food on the table instead
We have shrubs that bloom
With the changing seasons
Many are fragrant
And we grow them for that reason
Some plants are evergreen
Giving pleasure all year round
While a few are cut back
Each spring to the ground
We have a shady arbour
And a sun drenched patio
Are you getting the picture
Of this beautiful scenario?
It is wonderful to watch
The trees reaching for the sky
Our garden gives us endless pleasure
And we tend to it with pride

LIFE OBSERVATIONS

Control

I am a very ordered person
I like to be in control
I boss people about
And set them challenging goals
I would make a good sergeant major
And keep everyone in line
I wouldn't stand for any nonsense
From those simply wasting time
I like to run a tight ship
With lots of rules and regulations
Though nothing is written down
And there is no legislation
I am very manipulative
That is what other people say
But all I really want
Is to get my own way
Being in control
Is very hard work
It has its own pressures
And is not a job to shirk
If you were to ask me
Why are you a control freak?
I would probably tell you to shut up
And not to even speak!

A Terrible Tease

I put my hand over yours
And give it a gentle squeeze
I am here to reassure you
And put you at your ease

I know how to make you relax
I only want to please
I am here to put your smile back
And you know I am a terrible tease

I intend to make you laugh
And grin from ear to ear
I will make you forget your troubles
And cast away your fears

Are you ready to feel happy
Are you ready to feel joy?
For I know all the tricks in the book
They are just waiting to be deployed

In a Rush

Rush, rush, rush
Always in a hurry
No time to think
Except if it's to worry
I have been doing a balancing act
Juggling all the demands burdening me
My life has become a rat trap
That is plain to see
If any one part of my schedule
Were to breakdown or go awry
I would be completely flummoxed
And it would surely make me cry
Plus there often isn't enough time
To fit everything in
So there is an ever increasing backlog
And to me this is a terrible sin
It prays on my mind
Constantly niggling in the background
Adding to the stress
And making my problems compound
I am like a bottle of champagne
Shake me any more and I'll go pop
And when I do suddenly burst
It will be you who has to mop up
Every single drop

Stress

I am under pressure
I am feeling stressed
I have too many tasks
That need to be accomplished
Where will I find the time
To fit everything in?
Life is so hectic
I don't know where to begin
My body has reacted
By pumping out adrenalin and cortisol
To boost my energy levels
And help me take control
But this response
Also has a negative side
It makes me feel anxious
And all churned up inside
For short periods of time
This is okay
But I don't want it continuously
Every single day
If that starts to happen
It could make me ill
And I may have to resort to
Popping a few pills
Of course a perfect world
Would be entirely stress free
But then I would never get out bed
And nothing would be achieved

Feigned Illness

Have you ever feigned illness
And used this as an excuse
To get out of doing something you didn't like
Or because if you failed you would have too much to
lose?
I have done it many times
And the stories I concoct are very lame
Of course I am frightened I will be found out
But I still do it all the same
I guess it demonstrates a lack of confidence
And a lack of self belief
I do it for my own preservation
It is a stress avoidance technique

Emotions

We all express different emotions
To things that are happening around
It may be a reaction to other people
Or to something that we've found
We are sensitive to our environment
Especially to the weather
We smile when the sun is shining
But when it snows we really shiver
We all understand what it is like
To feel happy or just sad
But we can also feel angry
In contrast to being glad
Sometimes we may be annoyed
When others don't see our point of view
We may want to fight them
And a battle will ensue

We can become frustrated
When things aren't going right
The opposite to those magical times
When we are as high as a kite
Emotions are ruled by hormones
And chemicals in our brains
It is interesting to ponder
How can this make us all feel the same?

Genes

Life is a journey
A passage through space and time
During which we grow and flourish
According to an architectural design
We are born with a certain genetic blueprint
That shapes how we physically grow
It also affects the development of our brains
And predetermines what personality traits we follow
I would argue that
'Nature' is more important than 'Nurture'
And I believe that our genes are crucial
In how our life skills are procured
Of course our experiences still influence
What kind of people we become
But it is our inherent spirit that defines us
And keeps our thoughts forever young

Argument

I don't want to argue
I can see your point of view
But I still think I am right
And what I am saying rings true
You should imagine yourself in my shoes
I am the one who has to suffer
But when I challenge you
You just put up a defensive buffer
Can't we find some common ground
Where both of us can gain?
A place where your pride won't be wounded
And my sanity will be maintained
All I want is to kiss and make up
There must be a way to solve the equation
If not then I could call in a third party
And we could go to arbitration
Let us settle our differences
I want to be friends once more
Life is too short to waste time arguing
Shall we call it an amicable draw?

Divorce

At what point do you decide
That your marriage is not a bed of roses?
How far does it have to deteriorate?
How deep the cracks you are exposing?
At some point you fall out of love
Your relationship no longer holds its attraction
Little things start to annoy
And drive you to distraction
All your common ground has been lost
You don't enjoy just being together
The sunshine has gone from your life
Ahead only seems to be stormy weather
So you will have to bail out
Even though this is the most difficult course
But in the end you have to bite the bullet
And ask for a divorce

Working

Does my job define who I am?
What if I choose not to work even though I can?
Surely it doesn't make me a lesser person
I am still me that's for certain
Yet it is still frowned upon to be unemployed
Despite the fact it is sometimes a situation we can't
avoid
Having a job doesn't affect your character
Working doesn't make you superior
So say you were to win the pools
You would resign today unless you were a fool

The Grace of God

I don't know the people I meet in the street
They pass me by just out of reach
I don't know their names or who they are
To me they are total strangers
But I can read a lot from their expressions
It is easy to tell if their lives are being threatened
I can see the suffering and the pain
Together with all the worry and the strain
I would like to stop them in their tracks
And tell them to chill out and learn to relax
But they would not take kindly to my intervention
Even though I only have good intentions
They would say not to interfere
Pretending that their problems had disappeared
So I continue to walk on by
Telling myself that "There but for the grace of God go I"

God and Health

Each day I set out in my car
I don't need much petrol, I am not going far
Just far enough to reach the pharmacy
To collect my medicinal armoury
Why do I make these little trips?
God only knows but does God really exist?
Can he fix my problems tomorrow?
Please God help me with my sorrow
At night I tell him all my problems
In the hope that he may be able to solve them
He never gives me any direct advice
Rather he hands me four large dice
To roll on to the floor
Demonstrating that a life is a lottery and no more
God never gives me feelings of derision
But rather prompts me to make my own decisions
To find a place of peace with inner tranquillity
Somewhere private for trance like surreality
But what form will this higher deity take?
Who cares when it makes me feel so great

Life

Life is never going to be easy
It is always going to be a test
But sometimes the odds are stacked against you
And all you can do is your level best

Life is never going to be fair
Someone will always try to spoil your plans
But if you are well prepared
You can raise your game to meet demand

Life is never going to be fought
On a level playing field
You have to stand up for yourself
And demonstrate that you won't yield

Life is never going to be all fun and games
But if you look in the right place
You will find there are many worthwhile things
And these are the ideals you should chase

Life is never just about receiving
The real pleasure comes from the giving
We are all in this together
And we have to create a world we all can live in

Life is never going to be forever
A fact that cannot be denied
But since we are here we can make it better
Or at least we have to try

Heaven

Let me take you by the hand
Let me lead you to the promised land
I know the way because I have been before
It is a wonderful space we can explore
It is somewhere all your problems can be solved
And you can learn how the world revolves
The answers to all those difficult questions
Will appear trivial on reflection
Once you are there you won't want to return
There will be no reason as far as you are concerned
God has created this paradise
Where all your dreams can be realised
Come with me prepared to have your sins forgiven
Welcome to this place that I call heaven

Being Human

We are individual people
Yet part of the human race
Our bodies comprise arms and legs
Plus of course a face
But there is more to being human
Than initially meets the eye
Let me make it clear to you
Let me tell you why
We are sentient beings
And know just who we are
We realise we are conscious
Different from animals, machines or cars
Our minds operate on different levels
Including dreaming and being awake
We also need our deep sleep
Otherwise we can get in quite a state

173

There is a light within us
That burns so very bright
It joins us all together
A bond that's very tight
We know we all must die
This will happen to us one day
But do we disappear
When we pass away?
I would like to think that things continue
That this inner glow won't fade
In the end we'll become one with 'God'
Because we're 'heaven made'

Life and Death

The life we live is fragile
It could even end today
No one knows what is round the corner
And whether everything is going to be okay
Will I know when the time has come
For me to leave this world behind?
Will I get a premonition
Or some other warning sign?
The thought of death is chilling
Although I realise I am mortal
I believe there is another realm
And this life is merely a portal
My soul will make a transition
From my body into light
To become part of a higher deity
One that is pure and bright
All my sins will be forgiven
And my heart will find it's resting place
I won't be frightened
Because I know I won't be alone in outer space

Passing Away

I will never forget you
Even though you have passed away
I can still feel your presence
As I force myself to live another day
All the years we spent together
Are filed in my memory
They can never be erased
They will stay with me for all eternity
I come across little things
As I potter around the house
Things that remind me of you
And only you and I would know about
They are very comforting
When I am feeling lonely
Because I know that you are still watching
And you are trying to console me
One day we will be reunited
When God decides my life should end
But for now I still imagine you here
Or at least that's what I pretend

Death

Death
The ultimate transition
When our souls
Stretch out into oblivion

Constrained
By our bodies no more
Free to roam
Should we wish to explore

At Peace
The final resting place
A continuous dream
We can't escape

The End
Of our mortality
But let's pray it is the start
Of a new and fabulous journey

Our Father

The death of our Father
Is a terrible tragedy
It is hard to take in
It is hard to believe
He has been snatched from us
By a cruel twist of fate
And now we must take time
To remember and contemplate
He was a wonderful Dad
Someone on whom you could rely
He always gave more than he had
That cannot be denied

He loved us all
In his own special way
And we will miss him
Every single day
But we should not mourn
For his life was fulfilled
We should celebrate this man
Knowing that in death he loves us still

When

When I am ill
I am very restless
I can't sit still
Despite being listless

When I am down
My thoughts keep churning
Spiralling round
For the good times yearning

When I can't cope
I crave affection
Someone to instil hope
And give me direction

When I am well
I can put the world to right
Never wishing to break that spell
Soaring to those dizzy heights

When I am stable
I can give so much love
For I become enabled
Blessed by God above

Happiness

The feeling of happiness is difficult to define
It is an inner state that's so sublime
I know it can be easy to lose
Especially when my mind becomes sick or a little
confused

It is like the sweet scent of perfume
That can sometimes overwhelm or even consume
It is the warm glow of satisfaction
When a job's been worth doing on reflection

But all this evaporates when I become mentally ill
Where all my endeavours seem to come to nil
And once happiness is gone it is hard to get back
It is as if I have simply lost the knack

A monumental effort is required to make the sadness
go
And for happiness to return when I have been feeling
low
Rest assured I will savour every 'well' minute
I will relish the time and live it to the limit

More To Life

There must be more to life than work, work, work
So I am setting out to search, search, search
For a vocation that is fun, fun, fun
And will satisfy me when the day is done, done, done

I want to give, give, give
And show others how to live, live, live
In a way that protects their mental health, health, health
Which is more important than any wealth, wealth, wealth

Our time on this earth is so very short, short, short
And happiness cannot be bought, bought, bought
It is a skill that can be taught, taught, taught
It just requires a little thought, thought, thought

Redundancy

Nobody's job is safe
It can always be taken away
I have just been given my marching orders
So I won't be the one who stays

It is a slap in the face
A real good kick in the teeth
After all my loyal service
I am to be thrown on the scrap heap

I have been made redundant
Apparently my job has been axed
Other people will have to do my work
Because of economic cut backs

Naturally I am saddened
But I know I have much to proffer
I will find another niche
Where I can draw money into the coffers

I am hopeful of my prospects
I am not going to wallow in self pity
I acknowledge I may be in for a bumpy ride
But I believe one day I will be sitting pretty

New Job

I told you something would come along
I am back in the workplace where I belong
It should be an exciting time for me
But I view it rather apprehensively
In this job there will be new names and faces
To be remembered and assimilated
Then there will be all the papers to be compiled
Trying to make sure every thing is correctly filed
There will be so many things to learn
And to begin with I may not know which way to turn
So pray for me that I don't come unstuck
For I deserve a little piece of luck

Regret

As I lie awake at night I reminisce
And conjure up pictures of the past
There are many fond memories
But there are others that are in stark contrast

It is these sadder moments
That bring feelings of regret
Up until today I have not made them apparent
I have kept my thoughts secret

Now I feel it necessary
To get everything off my chest
I need to be unburdened of this weight I carry
Please listen while I confess

So many times I have let you down
By being engrossed with my own needs
You have every right to frown
That much I must concede

I should have given you more of me
I know I didn't help you enough
But I beg you to forgive me
For you are my one true love

Love and Money

Money makes the world go round
Well that's what I've been told
We are too materialistic
Constantly looking for things to have and hold
I find myself agreeing with that
For I often spend my money too quickly
I buy clothes, shoes and bric-a-brac
It really isn't very tricky
But I ask "Does this make us happy?"
To which my answer has to be "No"
All we need is the giving and receiving of love
That's what creates our inner glow
Money can't buy us these affections
They can't be made in a factory
Rather the capacity to love is in all of us
And we can give it out for free

Sharing and Caring

We live in a sheltered world
Protected from the elements
We are cocooned in out houses
Built of bricks and cement
However, we must remember
That many people live in poverty
Their lives are not a bed of roses
But we often fail to see
We don't want to accept
That there are so many who are suffering
And we really should take time to care
To show that it is our love we're offering
Our world would be a better place
If the wealth were shared around
So when the charity tins are rattled
Dig deep into your pocket for that last pound

My Brain

My brain is a very complex mass
Of neurones, glial cells and fat
Everything is linked together
In a way that's rather clever
It has the capacity to create
This personal world or inner state
My brain can organise all my thoughts
And wants continuously to be taught
It uses up lots of energy
Particularly when laying down new memory
And it has the ability to retrieve
Information I have previously received
But it can play tricks on me as well
Especially if I am mentally ill
The secret to my brain's success
Is that it is adaptable under stress
And this leads me to conclude
That my brain has real attitude

183

Your Brain

Is your brain stagnating
Through lack of stimulus?
Then I will give you some of my energy
Of which I have a surplus
Your brain needs lots of exercise
Every single day
Otherwise its capacity
Begins to drain away
Just how does your brain work?
How does it operate?
When electrical impulses
Are all it generates?
It is an interesting question
To which I don't have a reply
I can't start to answer it
And I won't begin to try
But what I do know is
Your brain is very versatile
It can alter according to the situation
And it can do it all in style

New Tricks

You can always teach an old dog new tricks
Our memory should never worsen with age
For even when our bodies give out
We have plenty of spare neurones for info storage
So we should not become forgetful
We just need to exercise our brains
Then the input we are given
Still has a chance to be retained
We remember pictures better than words
We are particularly good with the human face
Although putting names to them
May be difficult to place

184

For recalling text or literature
Key words are the solution
Then we just fill in the gaps
Avoiding any confusion
Of course we can still learn things off by heart
Like remembering our timetables by rote
Or maybe show off a little
By reciting a famous quote
If we look back at our lives
And dwell on what has passed
It is our fondest memories that spring to mind
Particularly those that made us laugh

Your Mind

What is on your mind?
What are you thinking about?
Is it something trivial
Or is it something with a little more clout?
It can be funny if you pause
And consciously listen to what your brain has to say
At times it may be concentrating on reality
At others it may be far away
For instance when you drive your car
And you are travelling from A to B
You suddenly find you have arrived
But you can't remember the bit in between
Your brain is multi-tasking
Doing many things at once
It is juggling several balls in the air
Without any one thought becoming ensconced
Your brain is very pliable
It can be moulded into different forms
We hope it never lets us down
And is always ready to perform
But whatever you are thinking
It is personal to you
Only you know what is happening
No one else can intrude

Ideas

I sit here at my desk
About to put my brain to the test
Can I have a bright idea
That will make me a millionaire?
I want to think of something clever
That will stay with me forever
It will have to make me proud
And a bit bigheaded if that's allowed
Perhaps it will be a new gadget
Or a cure for a disease that's tragic
Maybe I'll find a quick solution
For all this global pollution
Of course it could just be
A way to end abject poverty
There is no way of knowing
Exactly which direction I'll go in
For now I continue to rotate
All my thoughts at a tremendous rate
And pray that one day I'll succeed
In what I have set out to achieve

My Education

I can remember vividly
My first day at school
It was all a little bewildering
I didn't understand all the social rules
But I was quick to learn
About numbers and words
I loved doing adding up
And trying to spell new things I'd heard
As time went by
I acquired all the essential skills
Of how to write correctly
And work out the mathematics of a shopping bill
I moved on to the Secondary Level

186

Where the subjects were more demanding
And I tried to keep out of trouble
So as not to be given a reprimanding
I was very fortunate
In that I excelled at doing exams
I left school fully prepared
For the next step in my life plan
On to University then
My target an honours degree
This required more complex thinking
It really tested my ingenuity
After three years of study
You would have thought I'd have had enough
But I was a glutton for punishment
I pushed on for my doctorate
My brain was fully developed
The education process was complete
I was ready to face world out there
To stand on my own two fee

Unite

The children of the world must unite
Or soon this earth will not sustain life
We constantly pollute our atmosphere
That damages the ozone layer
This in turn leads to global warming
And then one day you will get up in the morning
To find the planet has been irrevocably damaged
All because our behaviour has been badly managed
There will be no going back
We will be stopped dead in our tracks
We will suffer the consequences
Unless we intervene and come to our senses
If we act now without delay
It is not too late for our world to be saved
We can create a bright future
By not putting the earth through any further torture

Trust and Truth

We trust that those who lead us
Are pure of heart and mind
We pray they don't abuse their power
And that their actions are not maligned
As children we look up to our elders
Having faith in what is said
And believing that we will be guided
Down the path of righteousness
But Beware!
For all may not be as it seems
There are people out there
Who will step on others to reach their dreams
We must not be manipulated
We must see through the front
Even though everything appears plausible
It may all just be a stunt
You never get something for nothing
So don't let yourself be duped
Make your own stand in the world
And always search for the truth

Sleep

I couldn't sleep last night
My brain would not keep still
My thoughts were uncontrollable
And my mind had it's own free will
I tried counting sheep
But that didn't help
So I turned to reading
A book from on the shelf
It was called 'The mind at Night'
And it made me realise
There is more to being asleep
Than I had initially surmised
We cycle between several states
From deep sleep through to dreaming
And to me it is this REM sleep time
That is the most intriguing
Our brains play different scenarios
Based on things we've fantasised
But we can't act them out
Because we are paralysed
What use is this dreaming?
Does it prepare us for the next day?
Or does it have some other function
Who can really say?
Apparently if you miss your REM sleep
On one particular night
The next time you go to sleep
Your brain tries to set the balance right
If I can't get to sleep then
I won't become irate
Because I know my mind is clever
And it will compensate

Bad Dreams

I need your arms to hold me tight
Especially in the middle of the night
When my dreams are full of woe
And I am lost for any place to go
My nightmares predict a gloomy future
Where I am about to fall down a narrow fissure
I long for you to rouse and wake me
So that the devil doesn't take me
But you are fast asleep by my side
And our two worlds don't coincide
Suddenly I sit up screaming
And I realise I have been dreaming
Even though I know it is all an illusion
A part of me believes in these intrusions
This is what scares me the most
As I sit here eating my morning toast
Wondering what is imagined and what is real
Fearing sleep for it has now lost its appeal

A Parents View of Sleepovers

It is Saturday night
It is sleepover time
How many friends are staying?
Is it eight or is it nine?
Girls with the girls
Boys with the boys
Fighting over the computers
Everyone wants their favourite toys
Playing the latest PC game
Or watching a DVD
They are all vying for the widescreen TV
Once that is settled
They start demanding food

All that junk stuff
Which is doing them no good
Then there is the difficult problem
What time to go to bed?
It is a delicate issue
And we must take care how we tread
In the end we let them get on with it
Trusting there will be no cause for alarm
After all we are under the same roof
So they can't really come to any harm

Migraine

What I am experiencing
Is something quite obscene
I have a pain inside my head
The sort that makes you want to scream
I have been hit by a migraine
It is more than just a headache
It is completely debilitating
And won't go away however hard I remonstrate
I feel sick to my stomach
The nausea comes and goes in waves
All I can do is lie in bed
With the curtains drawn to create a bit of shade
I would like to fall asleep
To avoid further suffering
In the hope I'll wake up
To find I am recovering
I have stopped eating chocolate
I have cut down on caffeine
On the assumption that these are the triggers
That are destabilising me
But whatever the cause of my migraine
There is no escaping the fact
They often strike from nowhere
And I dread the next attack

Growing Old

I don't want to grow old
And have to draw my pension
If I were to talk to God
Do you think he would grant me a life extension?
I don't want my hair to turn grey
Or see my body deteriorate
Because in my mind's eye
I am still only twenty eight
So I slap on anti wrinkle cream
And put make up on my face
In the vain hope
That the lines can be erased
I work out at the gym
To try to keep my muscles tight
I am careful what I eat
And I try to kerb my appetite
But the inevitable will happen
One day I will be old
Unless the scientists can develop drugs
That will put the aging process on hold

Bored

I am completely bored
Fed up to the back teeth
There is nothing I can think of
That will give me light relief
I try to listen to the radio
Or watch something on TV
But my attention span is short
And the programs just don't grab me
Reading a book is even harder
I can't focus on the words
It seems a pointless exercise
I know that sounds absurd

Naturally there are the chores
But these can be brushed aside
For they are unrewarding
And don't keep me satisfied
I would like to be creative
To draw or maybe paint
This would occupy me
Ridding me of my complaint
I am sure you can think
Of lots of things to do
So please let me know your secret
For I really haven't got a clue

Retail Therapy

When I am down or feeling kind of bored
I like to cheer myself up by having a reward
I like to go out on a shopping spree
And this what you would call 'Retail Therapy'
I don't have to have a specific item in mind
I just want to browse and see what I can find
Sometimes it is clothes other times it is shoes
When I see both together then it can become difficult to
choose
I also buy chocolate and cream cakes if I can
And I say 'Sod the diet. It can go down the pan'
Whatever I spend my money on, whatever I decide
It gives me a real buzz and makes me feel all warm
inside
If you don't understand what I am saying
Then you are probably too worried about who will be
paying
But if all the shops were to close then I don't know
what I would do
I would probably consult my lawyer and I would have to
sue!

Computers

Computers have come to rule our lives
Without them we would not survive
They are essential for passing information
Back and forth around the nation
They control the tiny incubator
That keeps alive babies who are premature
And they help the police solving crimes
Providing finger print data at the appropriate time
There are countless examples of their use
The list is endless and without refute
I look back to see how far we have come
Computers are so much more than playing games and
having fun

Ambition

Do you have an aim in life?
Do you have a burning ambition?
Maybe you would like to be a soldier
And fire off rounds of ammunition
Alternatively you might want to climb a mountain
Or dive down to the ocean floor
It could be that you want to parachute from a plane
Or even trek into the jungle's dark interior
This is the stuff dreams are made of
These are our fantasies
And if you are lucky enough to live them out
It results in pure ecstasy
Start forging ahead right now
To make sure your ambition is realised
And remember that you must be single minded
There is no room for compromise

Canoeing

I can feel another poem brewing
Let me tell you about canoeing
It was a sport I did in my youth
It was an obsession to tell the truth
I used to compete at the highest level
And it took me on many worldly travels
The boat I used was very slim
Just wide enough to squeeze my bottom in
When I dipped my paddles into the water
My boat and I would begin to surge forward
The canoe would push the water aside
But if I stopped I would continue to glide
At full speed the boat would almost hum
And a perfect experience really had begun
I used to train two or three times a day
And I did all this without any pay
Now I miss the satisfaction of being that fit
But who knows maybe one day I will go back to it

Tennis

Tennis is good exercise
For the young to the very old
It can be played in most weathers
Although you sometimes get quite cold
You use a racquet and a ball
That you hit very hard
And you compete on a rectangular court
Or in your own back yard
You can play by yourself or with a partner
It doesn't matter which
Tennis is very sociable
Both on and off the pitch
The scoring goes 15, 30, 40
Followed by game
But sometimes you go to deuce
Which can increase the strain
The match can involve love
At the very start
And you have to get at least 2 sets
Before you play the winning part
Tennis is a great sport
It uses all your muscles
But you also have to use you brain
And you can have some mental tussles
I do enjoy my Tennis
It gives me so much pleasure
Particularly when I am the champion
Those are the moments that I treasure
In my opinion Tennis is the best game
It really takes a lot of heart
It requires good coordination
But it's never too late to start!

Playing Tennis with Your Spouse

Playing tennis with your spouse
Should really knock the opposition out
Because you should be on the same wavelength
Giving your pairing extra strength
However it is not quite that straight forward
Being so close can make things awkward
You are less tolerant of your partner's mistakes
They annoy a little more, they aggravate
And when your spouse tries to tell you what to do
The words seem to cut right through
There are plusses of course
Like knowing exactly their position on the court
Also you don't get so tight on the big points
There is no fear that you will disappoint
And at the end of the game
Your memories of the match are the same
This means that later when you reflect
You can tell your story while your other half interjects

Exercise

I have lots of get up and go
I can't sit around and be a couch potato
I don't want to fall victim
To a failing cardiovascular system
I walk, play tennis and use the rowing machine
In pursuit of becoming a fitness queen
A number of years back
You would have found me on the running track
Or paddling my canoe down a stream
Striving to be the best but often taking things to
extreme
Now I only compete with myself
Improving both my physical and mental health
For your brain releases endorphins when exercising
Making you feel good without realising
Take a leaf out of my book
Give yourself a long hard look
You should take fitness seriously
As it has the added bonus that it can cure obesity

Competition

Why do we like to compete?
Why do we strive to achieve?
It is because we want to better ourselves
And reinforce our self belief
Also it is the thrill of competition
That gives us a real buzz
And satisfies a basic instinct
It is a feeling that we love
Our ancestors had to hunt for food
And face the perils involved
Whereas now we just sit at our desks
Letting the world revolve

Excitement is what we seek
Always testing our limitations
Wanting to demonstrate we are not weak
And that we deserve congratulations
But let us hope
We don't run out of steam
For this would be detrimental
It would damage our self esteem
The challenge is like a drug then
That is why we crave competition
It is a culmination of the training
Bringing everything to fruition

Relaxation

What do you do to relax?
Maybe you like watching a football match?
Personally I like to lie in the bath and soak
I try not to make it overly deep or I'll choke
I also enjoy the odd glass of wine
Which I sip outside in the sunshine
If it is hot I like to jump in the pool
Where I can splash about and act the fool
I find a massage can be very relaxing
Or playing sport if it's not too taxing
Sometimes I like to be a couch potato
And watch the tele or listen to the radio
Whatever activity I finally choose
I know I will benefit, I just can't lose

Lottery

Looking in my purse I find
I am down to my last pound
Shall I spend it on the lottery?
Or am I really too miserly?
Winning would open up all manner of
opportunities
It would transform the life I lead
I could give up work today
And go on a fabulous holiday
I could buy a bigger house
With a pool for me to splash about
I could afford a new sports car
Then I could become the next boy racer
But is this an unrealistic scenario?
Wouldn't I be better off saving my money for
tomorrow?
The chances of winning are very slim
They are one in several million
Of course if I am to claim my prize
I would actually have to buy a ticket and that would be
a surprise

My Car

I have a small coupe
With a fold down top
The engine is very responsive
But knows a red light means stop
Sometimes I drive too fast
And I break the speed limit
But I watch out for cameras
Because I don't want to drop myself in it
I like to cruise around
Especially on a sunny afternoon

I am in my own little world
And the car acts as my cocoon
I wash it at least once a week
Occasionally I give it a wax
I keep it topped up with oil
And make sure the tyres have adequate tracks
My car is my status symbol
It shows I have plenty of cash
I am a very proud owner
And I'll race you if you want to be thrashed

Decorating

There is a new room to decorate
It requires a design that is ornate
I am painting the walls in shades of peach
And I have had to buy various pots of each
Emulsioning the ceiling has made my neck ache
But it has to be done for goodness sake
I have selected the curtains already
And I will hang them from metal poles that are steady
The carpet is soft and in a terracotta style
It has a slight pattern woven into the pile
The wardrobes have mirror doors
And are fitted from ceiling to floor
I also have an antique dressing table
Where I will sit to make myself presentable
To finish the room off I am getting a new bed
This is especially for my husband to rest his weary
head
Now the project is nearing its completion
And I can step back and admire all my decoration

Holiday

My suitcase is full to bursting
I am excited and I can't wait to depart
I have my ticket clutched in my hand
The next stop is the airport
I am jet setting for my summer break
To a mediterranean island in the sun
I am going to let my hair down
And have some serious fun
The hotel is right on the beach
And my room has an enchanting ocean view
The sea is lapping gently on the shore
The waves are a shimmering blue
I can catch some rays on the terrace
Right next to the paradise pool
But if the sun starts to burn and I get too hot
Then I can slip into the water all soothing and cool
The food is deliciously appetising
There is really too much choice
But I'm not going to worry about over eating
Because my diet and I have called a truce
In the evening the entertainment is laid on
And usually you would find me wincing
But today the singers are exceptionally good
And even the magician is fairly convincing
The nightclub is the next port of call
My friends and I can party till dawn
I will dance and drink the hours away
And eventually crash into bed with a yawn
The next day it will start all over again
The process will be repeated
I am enjoying every minute
It is bloody brilliant to use an expletive
All too soon it is time to go home
I have had a fabulous holiday
I look extremely healthy with a deep tan
Which I expect will wash off in couple of days

Food

Every day seems to revolve around eating
There are three main meals that need completing
Then there are the snacks in between
Which I try to hide so as not to be seen
Of course the only person I am cheating is me
And I do care about how I am perceived
I try to eat food that is healthy
Therefore I have no real reason to be stealthy
I like potatoes, pasta and rice
With a selection of toppings that add a little spice
I also enjoy puddings and deserts
Of which I don't consume too much or it'll hurt
As you can see I love my food
But sometimes it makes me burp which is rude

Chocoholic

I am a chocoholic
My addiction needs feeding regularly
I can't go without for very long
Before I start acting peculiarly
Any form of chocolate will do
From a Mars bar to a solid block
It will satisfy my craving
Although I still prefer a selection box
I can consume vast quantities
I find that very easy
It doesn't seem to make me sick
However I do admit to sometimes feeling queasy
I dread to think
How many extra calories I ingest
But can I still squeeze into my clothes?
Well, I know this is the ultimate test
Chocolate, Chocolate, Chocolate
At Christmas and Easter too
These are my favourite times of year
When my behaviour can be excused
The rest of the time I try to ration myself
But worry that one day all the chocolate will be gone
Just the mere thought gives me the shivers
I don't think I could carry on

War

Why do we go to war?
Is it to settle some petty score?
All too often it involves a clash of religion
Or an argument over who owns a particular region
Sometimes troops are sent in to quash civil upheaval
Or to remove a dictator who is evil
Whatever the reason for the fighting
People will get hurt and it is very frightening
Shooting and bombs, aircraft and tanks
Soldiers in combat of all different ranks
Many will die and not make it home
They will leave their loved ones completely alone
Bloodshed and tears are an inevitable fact
Until there is victory or some sort of pact
But does war resolve the underlying conflicts?
Surely it is unnecessary and just a political trick

Terrorists

There are many millions of people
Who make up the world's population
And we as individuals
Only have contact with the smallest congregation
We all live together
In a complex society
Where there are unwritten codes of conduct
That allow us to integrate harmoniously
But there are a few
Who are hell bent on ruining it for others
They are a tiny minority
And often operate undercover
You would call them terrorists
And you must admire them for their persistence
Their sole purpose is to wreak havoc
They challenge our very existence
As a result there is a continuous battle
To stop their reproduction
And to ensure they cannot develop
Weapons of mass destruction
We must be vigilant
In keeping the terrorists at bay
Then we can expose them all
And bring them to account on judgement day

Siblings

Thank God I'm not an only child
For the weight of expectation would be too great
And although my parents are meek and mild
The pressure to succeed may have been too much to take

But it goes without saying
I always had to vie for attention
There was often squabbling
That shouldn't go without a mention

I wanted to be the best
To outshine the other three
But as an adult I tend to acquiesce
And recognise that our parents loved us equally

It is good to know your genes
Are shared with your siblings
Our family tree can now be screened
By the technology of DNA sequencing

This creates a blueprint that shows
Many traits are passed down in our ancestry
I just hope I don't follow
A streak of lunacy!

Being a Mum

Being a Mum
Is a job in its own right
Starting with all that crying
In the middle of the night
There are hungry mouths
And dirty nappies
It is a balancing act
Trying to keep everyone happy
The cooking and the washing
The ironing and the cleaning too
All must be fitted in
To the busy schedule
I also have to go to work
In order to make ends meet
And to enable us to afford
Those little extra treats
Don't forget love and affection
Must still be shared around
Catering for emotional needs
And keeping the family safe and sound
Please remember also
That Mums can never be ill
Because the world would cease to turn
It would come to a complete standstill

Friends

I have lots of friends
Dotted around the world
They include recent acquaintances
And those I met when I was a girl
My friends come from
All walks of life
And a few I only know
Because they are someone's husband or wife
My colleagues I see every day
When we are working hard
Others I only keep in touch with
Via a Christmas card
But no matter whether we are
Close or miles apart
Each friend has
A special place in my heart
The telephone helps me keep in touch
With those far away
And I always promise
That I will visit them one day
There are one or two people
With whom I have a very tight friendship
We couldn't live without each other
We are joined at the hip
You can't choose your family
But you can choose your friends
And I hope they will standby me
Even if I go round the bend

Long Time, No See

It is so good to see you
It has been such a long time
Why didn't we keep in touch
Or just drop each other a line?
A lot of water has passed
Under the proverbial bridge
But we still think on the same wavelength
As if our friendship was just on ice in the fridge
Let's celebrate our re-established bond
Let's make up for those missed years
Look I have a bottle of champagne waiting
All we need to say is "Cheers"

A Friend in Need

My daughter has a friend in need
She is about to move to the Outer Hebrides
Naturally she doesn't want to go
She would prefer to stay with the friends she knows
Her parents don't seem to have taken
Her feelings into consideration
I guess they want to escape
From this interminable rat race
There has been no discussion
There has only been a unilateral decision
In an ideal world the friend could live here
Because this girl is no trouble and is very dear
All we can do is comfort her when she cries
And tell her she will still be part of our lives
She can visit in the holidays
But in the meantime she will just have to be brave

Friends like These

Why do I need enemies?
When I have friends like these
They say one thing to your face
And stab you in the back with consummate ease
When they want to borrow something
They rush around without a thought
But never bring the item back
It doesn't occur to them it had to be bought
'Lend us a fiver
No better make it ten
I promise I will pay you back
When my next dole cheque comes in
But I never see the money
I never expected I would
Because these people have no conscience
They don't realise it is possible to be kind and good

Talent

Some people have a talent
Or a creative streak
Maybe they are good with words
And know just how to speak
Others express themselves through art
And are clever with their hands
They use many different mediums
From paint to clay or even sand
Gardeners grow plants
And the best we call 'green fingered'
These people often talk to their flowers
Or play them songs by well known singers
Musicians play their instruments
And that is their special gift
Or as a teacher you can inspire others
And give them such a lift

Many people channel their energy
Into playing sport
They want to be the champion
But don't forget that they were taught
Having a talent is exciting
And is something to be shared
It gives you satisfaction
Right deep down in there

Addiction

What is your poison?
What do you take when you are in need?
Do you hit the bottle?
Or do you swallow some ecstasy?
Whatever form your escape mechanism takes
Watch out because you can become a victim
Where you start to rely on this behaviour
It has turned into an addiction
Initially you may be unaware
That you have a problem at all
But your coping strategy has backfired on you
And your emotional prop has become evil
It is a habit you have got into
It has become a way of life
To break the pattern is very difficult
But here is some sound advice
Everyday there is the chance
To start with a clean slate
Tomorrow you have the potential to stop
The time for giving up will never be too late

Doctor

You are my doctor, you are my friend
On your sound advice I can depend
I can come to you any time I like
Even in the middle of the night
When I need you, you are always there
And I would like to thank you for your continued care
I know that I can be difficult to help
But when I am ill I can't look after myself
I value your judgement and your reassurance
And I know that sometimes I test your endurance
But your knowledge and understanding are deeply
respected
And you do everything that I would have expected
I am very lucky to have you as my GP
Your service really is of the highest quality!

My Doctor

Thank you for being there
Thank you for your all your care
I am indebted to you
And would like to show my gratitude
You always greet me with a smile
You have a special welcoming style
I trust your judgement and expertise
And when it is time for me to leave
I am completely reassured
That all the avenues have been explored
Thank you again for everything you have done
Just seeing you is often half the battle won

Middle Age Spread

I have become a victim of middle age spread
Something that I always viewed with fear and dread
I would rather be somewhere else instead
But maybe this is what was intended

Maybe I was destined to be overweight
Maybe I was supposed to be this shape
It is a situation that I really hate
But maybe I will have to accept it with good grace

For I am driving myself into the ground
Constantly looking for ways to shed a few pounds
All the diets are never as good as they sound
They have all defeated me in the last round

I will have to buy clothes for the fuller figure
And find things that still flatter
I will have to embrace the bigger picture
And stop putting myself through any further torture

Overweight

I am over weight
Too heavy for my height
It really is a problem
And it's something I don't like
I have tried dieting
But that doesn't seem to help
I don't have enough will power
And I can't control myself
The medication that I take
Doesn't improve the situation
In fact I'm sure it leads
To an exacerbation
I haven't given up though
Because I am not happy with how I am
And I will watch the media closely
For the next dieting scam

Mobile Phone

In our modern world
Mobile phones reign supreme
We can't do without them
They are indispensable or so it seems
They are useful in emergencies
For example when your car breaks down
We also use them in the situation
When someone needs to be found
Mobile phones help us coordinate
Our busy and hectic lives
And we can constantly keep in touch
With our husbands or wives

215

Just how did we manage
Not so many years ago?
The techno revolution has been rapid
And it is still in full flow
I keep my mobile in my pocket
It vibrates when there's a call
But I must remember to turn it off
When I'm at the school recital

An Easter Thought

Christ died to save us from our sins
He was hammered onto a cross with pins
This must have created intense pain
A barbaric act ordered by someone insane
But the scriptures told us this was not the end
Jesus rose from the dead, he did ascend
Into heaven to be with his father
And to care for mankind forever after
Easter then should be a day of celebration
A time to praise the Lord and give him exaltation

Christmas is Coming

Christmas is coming
My goose is already fat
The old man is in a home
So he won't need any money in his hat
The choir is at the door
And they are ready to sing
The children are excited
About what Santa will bring
But they will only get toys in their stockings
If they still believe
This is the magic of Christmas
It is a time when dreams become reality
We all hope it snows
To make the scene all frosty and bright
As we gather round the tree
To watch the decorations twinkle by candle light
There is a present for everyone
Hopefully they will all get a surprise
If there are too many chocolates
Then our New Year's resolution will be exercise!

Christmas

Christmas comes but once a year
Thank God because the expense is dear
The shops must really rake it in
And most of the stuff will end up in the bin
We buy enough food to last a month
And go to the supermarket more than once
Then we eat and drink like there is no tomorrow
Forgetting how the hangover will cause so much
sorrow
But the children will have such tremendous fun
Christmas is always special when you are young

Of course the littlest children often prefer the box
And we quickly discard the obligatory pair of socks
But there is a message behind all the celebrations
It was when Jesus was born for our salvation
We must remember this important fact
Because for some it will make up for the presents they
lack
We are the lucky ones here at home
So please give a thought for those who spend
Christmas alone

Christmas Time

Christmas is the time of year
When everyone is in good cheer
All our problems are cast aside
And together we celebrate Yuletide
There will be ample food and drink
But we try hard not to be chained to the kitchen sink
The preparations put us in high spirits
And we endeavour not to consume alcohol above the
legal limit
Gifts are bought for our friends and family
They are scattered beneath the tree
We hope everyone receives their hearts desire
Because this year the shopping has been inspired
That leads to one final thought
Make sure you don't spent more than you ought!

A Message to my Children at Christmas Time

Santa has decided that
You are too old for a stocking
I break this news gently
So that it is not too shocking
You have worked out
That Santa is an alias for Mum
And all the trickery of previous years
Was just a bit of fun
But don't let it spoil
The magic of Christmas Time
You will still get lots of surprises
Unless you have committed a dastardly crime
Santa has been working hard
During the build up to the festivities
To try to make everything exciting
And more than just the Nativity
Santa wants you to get involved
To soak up the atmosphere
And hopes you have a Merry Christmas
Followed by a Happy New Year

New Year's Resolution

My New Year's Resolution
Is to go on a slimming diet
I will cut out fatty foods
And all the trips to the fridge on the quiet
I will reduce my calorific intake
And try to do more exercise
I need to shed a few pounds
In order to go down in dress size
All this excess fat I am carrying
Needs to be disbursed
I am sure that I can do it
And I am prepared that it may hurt
But I know it is down to will power
I have to strengthen my resolve
If I am to achieve my goal
Then a little hard work is involved
Let's come back in a years time
To see if I have succeeded
I hope that I will be seen in different light
And that I can squeeze back into that yellow polka dot
bikini

CONCLUDING REMARKS

A Self Fulfilling Prophecy

Do you believe in superstition?
Do you believe fate put you in this position?
Do you believe in destiny?
Do you believe your life is a self fulfilling prophecy?

Because if you do it means you can't change
Because if you do your world can't be rearranged
Because if you do then you have no control
And it is already determined whether you will reach
your goals

I don't think this is the case
I think things can be altered or erased
I think we can manipulate our circumstances
To create our own opportunities and chances

All we have to do is have a positive frame of mind
All we have to do is picture ourselves as part of a
grand design
All we have to do is be instinctive
And in this way we make our lives distinctive

My Solace

My writing is my solace
It allows my true expression
The words are chosen carefully
To give the right impression
I can pour out my feelings
I can bare my soul
The content reflects my mood
Which can take it's emotional toll
But it is better to get everything out
Than try to bottle it up inside
And the total release I feel
Cannot be described
When I record my feelings
My brain shifts to a higher gear
All my thoughts are elevated
And my thinking becomes clear
I say again my writing is my solace
It is my form of escape
It is of great comfort
And defies all time and space

Epitaph

If you were to write my epitaph
It would have to make everyone laugh
Because despite of my depressive illness
I don't live in a world that is entirely humourless
I like to lark about and have a joke
Just as much as the next bloke
But my epitaph would also have to say
That I did everything in my own way
I live my life according to an unwritten code
A creed that keeps me on the straight and narrow
It sets high moral standards
But to abide by it isn't all that hard

And I would like to be remembered
For my kind and caring nature
I try to give more than I take
I am a selfless person and that's deliberate
Please record I am intelligent too
And I did my bit in the search for truth
Finally I give my all in what life throws my direction
And I love all mankind without exception

Magic

I can be pathetic
I can even be apathetic
At times I need to be sympathetic
Especially when things happen that are tragic

But I can also be electric
A sort of energy conduit
I have an inner power to be specific
A quality that is quite intrinsic

In reading this book I trust you have heard the sweet
music
That makes me tick and feel terrific
That inspires me and makes my life graphic
I hope I have touched you with my special kind of
magic

Round and Full

My life is round and full
And I am cared for by gentle people
My family and friends play their part
Although the professionals were key at the start
To begin with I was observed around the clock,
Which came as quite as an unnerving shock
Even in the middle of the night
They checked to see if I was alright
Slowly but surely I grew stronger
I didn't need constant supervision any longer
I was learning how to manage
There had been no irrevocable damage
With time, medication and support
I was able to re-gather my thoughts
Today I receive care in the community
But there is always back up in an emergency
I have my drugs working to their optimal
So the bad days have become quite exceptional
Now I can even help others in the same position
Guiding them in the right direction

Catastrophe

Is being mentally ill such a catastrophe?
Or can some good come of this apparent tragedy?
If I look back I can see it has changed my personality
And it has altered my perspective of the world quite
dramatically

I now think about my problems more rationally
When things go wrong I view it more philosophically
When good happens I see it more appreciatively
And I no longer do or say things so hypocritically

I am not driven to achieve constantly
Everything doesn't have to be done perfectly
Tasks don't have to be carried out with pinpoint
accuracy
A balance has been reached, I am in harmony

I now see caring for others as a higher priority
I want to help them to have a life of better quality
I have stopped questioning my own capabilities
And I have become a better person undoubtedly

Summary

I don't know what to write
The ink has dried up and my brain is on strike
This means you won't be hearing from me again
So I can put away the paper and discard my pen
Everything can return to normality
I can cease with this cerebral activity
I know that some of it has been disturbing
And even ultimately quite perturbing
But other parts have been light hearted
That was my intention when I first started
Don't be too disappointed as I take my leave
I expect in some ways you are rather relieved
I hope you have enjoyed what I have written
Because for me it has fulfilled my life long ambition
If you had told me that I could create a book
I wouldn't have believed I had what it took
But the proof is here for everyone to see
All that is left is to say thank you for listening to me